An Aid to Radiology for the MRCP

K. K. Ray BSc, MRCP

BHF Junior Research Fellow
Clinical Sciences Centre
Northern General Hospital
Sheffield
(formerly Walsgrave
Hospital NHS Trust, Coventry)

R. E. J. Ryder MD, FRCP

Consultant Physician
Department of Diabetes and Endocrinology
City Hospital NHS Trust
Birmingham

R.M. Wellings FRCS, FRCR

Consultant Radiologist
Department of Radiology
Walsgrave Hospital NHS Trust
Coventry

**Blackwell
Science**

Seventy per cent of the royalties from this book
will be donated to charities in Calcutta

© 2000
Blackwell Science Ltd
Editorial Offices:
Osney Mead, Oxford OX2 0EL
25 John Street, London WC1N 2BL
23 Ainslie Place, Edinburgh EH3 6AJ
350 Main Street, Malden
  MA 02148-5018, USA
54 University Street, Carlton
  Victoria 3053, Australia
10, rue Casimir Delavigne
  75006 Paris, France

Other Editorial Offices:
Blackwell Wissenschafts-Verlag GmbH
Kurfürstendamm 57
10707 Berlin, Germany

Blackwell Science KK
MG Kodenmacho Building
7–10 Kodenmacho Nihombashi
Chuo-ku, Tokyo 104, Japan

First published 2000

Set by Excel Typesetters Co., Hong Kong
Printed and bound in Great Britain at the
Alden Press Ltd, Oxford and
Northampton

The Blackwell Science logo is a
trade mark of Blackwell Science Ltd,
registered at the United Kingdom
Trade Marks Registry

For further information on
Blackwell Science, visit our website:
www.blackwell-science.com

DISTRIBUTORS

  Marston Book Services Ltd
  PO Box 269
  Abingdon, Oxon OX14 4YN
  (*Orders*: Tel: 01235 465500
           Fax: 01235 465555)

USA
  Blackwell Science, Inc.
  Commerce Place
  350 Main Street
  Malden, MA 02148-5018
  (*Orders*: Tel: 800 759 6102
           781 388 8250
       Fax: 781 388 8255)

Canada
  Login Brothers Book Company
  324 Saulteaux Crescent
  Winnipeg, Manitoba R3J 3T2
  (*Orders*: Tel: 204 837 2987)

Australia
  Blackwell Science Pty Ltd
  54 University Street
  Carlton, Victoria 3053
  (*Orders*: Tel: 3 9347 0300
           Fax: 3 9347 5001)

A catalogue record for this title
is available from the British Library

ISBN 0-632-04912-X

Library of Congress
Cataloging-in-publication Data

Ray, K. K., MRCP.
   An aid to radiology for the MRCP /
   K. K. Ray, R. E. J. Ryder,
   and R. M. Wellings
        p.   cm.
   Includes index.
   ISBN 0-632-04912-X
   1. Diagnosis, Radioscopic —
Examinations, questions, etc.
I. Ryder, R. E. J. (Robert Elford John)
II. Title.
   [DNLM: 1. Radiology examination
questions.   WN 18.2 R263a 1999]
RC78.15.R39   1999
616.07′57′076 — dc21
DNLM/DLC
for Library of Congress   98-51790
                                       CIP

An Aid to Radiology
for the MRCP

To my wonderful mother Ruby, for her hard work, sacrifice and unselfish dedication to her family. Her smile remains my inspiration.
&
To my father Kartik whose own achievements have been a constant example to me of the rewards of hard work and dedication.

Kausik K. Ray

Contents

Questions

Answers

Preface

The essence of medicine lies in the diagnosis and treatment of various conditions. The clinical diagnosis relies on many variables, one of the most important of which is the physician's ability to interpret various investigations. Modern radiology has become one of the most important diagnostic tools and is fundamental to the physician's knowledge.

This book is designed to mimic the format of the Member of the Royal College of Physicians (MRCP) exam, with a case history or stem being followed by a radiological test and a short answer section. Readers are asked to describe the radiological findings in each case. Good-quality images and the labelling of the abnormal findings on the original images should enable readers to convince themselves about specific radiological abnormalities, instead of having to guess where the abnormality lies. Further, the signs shown are listed to aid the speed of learning. Each case is linked to a short answer section that provides background knowledge. This is not meant to be comprehensive, but merely to whet the appetite for further reading. The book has been divided into eight general sections, so that readers can identify specific systems quickly. This book is intended to be a companion to Ryder, Mir & Freeman's *An Aid to Short Cases for the MRCP* (Blackwell Science).

The words of Robert Frost, 'But I have promises to keep, And miles to go before I sleep' seem to apply to most candidates sitting the MRCP exam. Those of us who have sat the exam are familiar with the lack of sleep during those stressful months and the promise to ourselves of better things to come. I hope that by writing this book we will help other doctors keep those promises and shorten the journey until they sleep!

Acknowledgements

We would like to thank Dr David Beale, Dr William Shatwell, Dr Tom Goodfellow, Dr Allison Duncan, Dr K. H. Sherlala and Dr John Chandy (Radiology Department of Walsgrave Hospital, Coventry) and Dr David Taylor (Department of Clinical Physics, Walsgrave Hospital, Coventry) for their contributions to the images shown in this book. Our thanks also go to Dr John Wingate (Department of Radiology, City Hospital, Birmingham), Dr David Carruthers (Lecturer in Rheumatology, City Hospital, Birmingham) and Mr Peter Ryan and Mr David Arkell (Consultant Urologists, City Hospital, Birmingham) for providing some of the images shown.

We are grateful to International Medical MultiMedia Ltd (14–16 Foxcombe Court, Abingdon Business Park, Abingdon, Oxon) for allowing us to use images from their extensive database. These images have been collected over the years by Dr Philip Gishen at King's College Hospital (London), and our thanks go to him for allowing us to publish his images.

We are indebted to our panel of expert reviewers in each speciality: Dr Peter Clarkson (Cardiology), Dr R. E. J. Ryder (Endocrinology), Dr Tariq Iqbal (Gastroenterology), Dr David Bareford (Haematology), Dr Edward Burton (Neurology), Dr Wajid Ayub (Nephrology), Dr Harmesh Moudgil (Respiratory Medicine) and Dr Deva Situnayake (Rheumatology).

We are grateful to Mrs Denize Gaitanoglou, Miss Marie Brolly and Mrs Kathryn Garas for their contribution to collecting the above cases and to Mr David Antrum for his help and encouragement throughout this venture.

Abbreviations

ACE	angiotensin-converting enzyme
ACTH	adrenocorticotrophic hormone
AF	atrial fibrillation
αFP	alpha-fetoprotein
AIDS	acquired immunodeficiency syndrome
ALT	alanine transaminase
ANA	antinuclear antibody
A–P	anteroposterior
APTT	activated partial thromboplastin time
ASD	atrial septal defect
AST	aspartate transaminase
AVM	arteriovenous malformation
AXR	abdominal X-ray
Ba	barium
Ca	calcium
c-ANCA	cytoplasmic antineutrophil cytoplasmic antibody
CMV	cytomegalovirus
COAD	chronic obstructive airway disease
COPD	chronic obstructive pulmonary disease
CREST	calcinosis, Raynaud's phenomenon, oesophageal involvement, sclerodactyly, and telangiectasia
CRP	C-reactive protein
CT	computed tomography, computed tomogram
CVS	cardiovascular system
CXR	chest X-ray
DDAVP	desmopressin (1-deamino-8-D-arginine vasopressin)
DMSA	dimercaptosuccinic acid
DSA	digital subtraction angiography
DTPA	diethylenetriaminepentaacetic acid
ECG	electrocardiography, electrocardiogram
EEG	electroencephalography, electroencephalogram
EMG	electromyography, electromyogram
ERCP	endoscopic retrograde cholangiopancreatography
ESR	erythrocyte sedimentation rate
ESWL	extracorporeal shock-wave lithotripsy
FBC	full blood count

Fe	iron
FNA	fine-needle aspiration
Hb	haemoglobin
HDL	high-density lipoprotein
HLA	human leucocyte antigen
HPOA	hypertrophic pulmonary osteoarthropathy
IGF	insulin-like growth factor
IgG	immunoglobulin G
IL	interleukin
IV	intravenous
IVU	intravenous urogram
K	potassium
LA	left atrium
LFTs	liver function tests
LH	luteinizing hormone
LHRH	luteinizing hormone-releasing hormone
LMN	lower motor neurone
LV	left ventricular, left ventricle
LVH	left ventricular hypertrophy
MAG3	mercaptoacetyltriglycine
MCV	mean corpuscular volume
MDP	methylene diphosphonate (disodium medronate)
MEN	multiple endocrine neoplasia
MIBI	methoxyisobutylisonitrile
mmHg	millimetre of mercury
MR	mitral regurgitation
MRA	magnetic resonance angiography
MRI	magnetic resonance imaging
Na	sodium
NSAIDs	non-steroidal anti-inflammatory drugs
OGTT	oral glucose tolerance test
P–A	posteroanterior
PAN	polyarteritis nodosa
p-ANCA	perinuclear antineutrophil cytoplasmic antibody
PBC	primary biliary cirrhosis
PCNL	percutaneous nephrolithotomy
PKD	polycystic kidney disease
PLT	platelet
PMH	past medical history
PO_4	phosphate
PT	prothrombin time

PTH	parathyroid hormone
RA	right atrium
RAS	renin–angiotensin system
RBBB	right bundle-branch block
RhA	rheumatoid arthritis
RLL	right lower lobe
RML	right middle lobe
RTA	renal tubular acidosis
SAARDs	slow-acting antirheumatoid drugs
SLE	systemic lupus erythematosus
SOB	shortness of breath
T_4	thyroxine
TB	tuberculosis
Tc	technetium
TIA	transient ischaemic attack
TIBC	total iron-binding capacity
TPHA	*Treponema pallidum* haemagglutination test
TSH	thyroid-stimulating hormone
TURP	transurethral resection of the prostate
UC	ulcerative colitis
UMN	upper motor neurone
US	ultrasound
UTI	urinary tract infection
V/Q	ventilation–perfusion
VDRL	venereal disease research laboratory test
WBC	white blood cell count
WCC	white cell count
ZE	Zollinger–Ellison syndrome

Introduction

Dr R.M. Wellings

When interpreting diagnostic images it is essential that a systematic and comprehensive approach is used. In this short introduction it is not possible to describe all the diagnoses you may meet, both in the examination and in your clinical work. Instead, some basic schemes are given to help you look at radiological images and see the information contained within them. These schemes are not intended to be regarded as the best and only way, but rather as an aid to your revision.

In the examination a structured approach to the questions will help minimize the impact of exam nerves:

1 The image presented to you and the information contained in the question *do* contain sufficient information to answer the question. Read carefully the question and the details given about the patient—particularly the history—and any findings should point you towards certain differential diagnoses.

2 Consider what kind of study you are being shown. The type chosen—for example, X-ray, ultrasound scan, computed tomogram (CT) or nuclear medicine—will be a strong clue as to the probable diagnosis. The more sophisticated the study, the more precise the information contained in the image. For example, chest pain and shortness of breath in combination with a ventilation–perfusion study are likely to relate to a pulmonary embolus in some way.

3 Use a systematic technique for analysing the image to look for important positive and negative features suggested by the history. Look for features of the conditions on your differential diagnostic list: do not just hope that the signs will make themselves known to you. Unlike textbooks, exam cases and real patients do not have helpful arrows appended to their images.

Plain radiography

Plain X-rays may show limited evidence of pathology and the signs may be subtle. You will be expected to be reasonably competent at assessing these as they will form a large part of your normal work. With plain X-rays, clues given in the text will be the critical guide in your search for the signs.

Chest

A chest X-ray (CXR) is such a ubiquitous part of clinical life it is inevitable that at least one or more cases will be based on it. The key is to look in a planned way, not desperately searching for clues.

To ensure that you look at all the elements of the CXR, we would recommend following a pattern similar to the one shown below:

1 Start at the heart and mediastinum.

2 Then move to the hila, lungs, bones, behind the heart and the review areas.

3 Then check the apices, the costophrenic recesses, the soft tissues on the film, the root of the neck and the area below the diaphragm.

4 In each area, key features must be assessed, as shown below.

Heart

Size:	is the film posteroanterior (P–A) or anteroposterior (A–P)?
Shape:	is there evidence of single- or multiple-chamber enlargement?
Position:	is it being pulled by fibrosis or collapse, or pushed by a pneumothorax or mass?
Calcification:	where is it? Pericardial or valvular?

Mediastinum

Size:	any widening? If so, in which part of the mediastinum?
Shape:	is there evidence of a mass?
Position:	is it being pulled by fibrosis or collapse, or pushed by a pneumothorax or mass?

Hila

Size and shape:	normally concave. Is there a mass, lymph nodes or abnormal vessels?
Position:	the left should lie above the right. In particular, this may be the most conspicuous cue for left lower lobe collapse.

Lungs. Compare the two lungs by looking at each side in turn and comparing it with the matching area on the other side. Work down until the whole area has been assessed (see Fig. 1.1).

Differences between two areas suggest either more air in the darker side—e.g. pneumothorax or decreased overlying soft tissue (mastectomy?), or an increased density in the lighter side (consolidation, mass, or fluid).

In an area of increased density, look to see if this corresponds to a known anatomical pattern, either intrathoracic (lobe, segment, pleural space) or extrathoracic (e.g. breast or muscle). If it does not, is the mass discrete or poorly defined? Is it single or multiple? Is there calcification? Is it in the lung or in the ribs?

Abdomen

Again, a coherent viewing strategy will aid you in the interpretation. There are certain key elements to look for. The bowel is best seen where it contains gas; other organs can be seen where the surrounding fat delineates their boundary sufficiently (this is normally the kidneys, the posterior aspect of the liver and the psoas muscles). Blurring of these outlines can be pathological in inflammatory conditions, but it is an unreliable sign obscured by many factors.

Gas. Check the pattern of gas within the abdomen. This should be within the bowel lumen: beware of gas in the wall in necrosis or pneumatosis intestinalis. The large bowel lies around the periphery of the abdomen, and normally shows haustral indentations. The small bowel is more central, and shows mucosal folds across its full width. Dilatation of bowel may indicate obstruction or may simply be gaseous. Loops over 2.5 cm are considered to be dilated. In situations in which there is clinical evidence of obstruction, you must remember that fluid-filled loops will not be

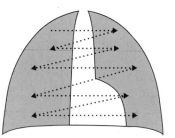

Figure 1.1 Scheme for viewing lungs.

seen on a plain film. Free gas in the peritoneum in perforation can be seen outside the bowel. The most sensitive examination for detecting this is the erect CXR. However, not all perforations release air into the peritoneum.

Calcium. The bones of the spine and pelvis may show pathology. Look for calcified stones in the kidney and renal tract; 10% of gallstones and 80% of renal stones are radiopaque. Check for calcification in the parenchyma of the abdominal organs. For example, the pancreas in chronic pancreatitis and the kidneys in nephrocalcinosis may be a key finding. Also look for calcification in aneurysmal vessels, tumour and parasitic conditions.

Contrast studies of the gastrointestinal tract

The poor demonstration of the bowel on the plain X-ray led to the introduction of contrast materials, normally substances containing barium or iodine, which delineate the lumen of the bowel with radiodense material and demonstrate stenoses and other pathologies.

Barium swallow

This study investigates the oesophagus and pharynx. Look for:
Stenoses, benign or malignant
Ulceration, peptic or infective
Pouches, pulsion or traction

Barium meal

This study investigates the oesophagus, stomach, duodenal cap and loop. This has largely been replaced by endoscopy. Malignancy must be suspected in gastric ulcers >2 cm across, but it is advisable to obtain histology on all gastric ulcers. Duodenal ulceration may indicate peptic disease or Crohn's disease.

Follow-through or small-bowel enema

This study investigates the small-bowel anatomy from the duodenum through to the colon. Transit time can be significantly extended by dysmotility conditions. The study allows detailed assessment of the mucosa for ulceration, thickening and masses, Crohn's disease, coeliac disease and malabsorption. These investigations may also demonstrate the level of stenosis or obstruction.

Barium enema

This demonstrates the anatomy of the colon, mucosal ulceration, stenoses, and polyps. The definition is not as good as in colonoscopy, but the facilities are more widely available. The terminal ileum can be demonstrated well on the barium enema, but this is dependent on reflux through the ileocaecal valve.

Urogenital radiography

The major study here is the intravenous urogram (IVU), which demonstrates the upper tracts and bladder. It is a good way of checking for stones, but the two-dimensional characteristics of the examination mean that large renal masses can be missed if they are not in profile on the renal margin. It is important to check for negative filling defects, tumours, or stones. Also check for any delay in drainage. The IVU is not a good measure of renal function, as it is influenced by too many factors for it to be reliable.

The plain X-ray can show stones or calcification in the kidneys, ureters, bladder, uterus and ovaries in tumorous and non-tumorous conditions.

Plain radiography of the peripheral skeleton and spine

The key issues here can be summed up using the mnemonic ABCDS:

Alignment.
Bone density.
Cartilage thickness.
Distribution.
Symmetry.

The pattern of changes is often critical in indicating a likely diagnosis:

Does the process involve large or small joints? Is there also involvement of the spine?
Is the bone matrix affected either globally or locally?

Is there decreased or increased bone matrix?

Are the joint spaces widened or narrowed? Is there effusion or cartilage loss?

Is the joint stable? Look for flexion and extension movement.

Is there evidence of erosion? Which joints are involved?

Is there any ligamentous or soft-tissue calcification? Ankylosing spondylitis, scleroderma?

Is there soft-tissue increase indicating swelling or increased bulk? For example, heel pad in acromegaly?

A similar process can be used in the spine, as the spine can be regarded as a complex stack of joints, vertebral discs and facets.

Angiography

This technique includes cardiac studies of the coronary vessels to demonstrate stenoses in coronary artery disease; and ventricular studies for valvular dysfunction, which can demonstrate stenosis of the valve (seen as a narrow jet in systole) or incompetence (with contrast entering a cardiac chamber against the normal direction of physiological flow).

In the peripheral setting, aneurysms of the aorta may be seen. The majority of conditions are manifested as stenoses or occlusions of vessels in atheromatous disease. However, systemic medical conditions such as polyarteritis nodosa (PAN) can manifest as microaneurysms in the renal or mesenteric system. Look for renal artery stenosis in hypertensive patients or those with poor renal function who are receiving antihypertensive medication. Fibromuscular hyperplasia shows a beaded pattern in the renal arteries distal to the renal origin.

The carotid is now generally investigated non-invasively with ultrasound, computed tomography (CT), or magnetic resonance imaging (MRI), but angiography is still the gold standard for carotid stenoses, and it remains the standard in demonstrating intracranial vascular problems, including intracranial aneurysms and arteriovenous malformations in subarachnoid haemorrhage.

Ultrasound

This commonly used modality has replaced many older techniques, and is used in every area of the body. It uses the transmission of sound through the body to create the image; air and bone, which reflect the sound, therefore act as major obstacles in the assessment of certain organs. For example, the adult brain is not accessible for ultrasound, because the skull is complete. In a baby, however, the fontanelles allow views to be obtained. Similarly, the lungs in their normal aerated state cannot be assessed with ultrasound, and bowel is poorly seen because of the gas it contains.

The advent of Doppler and colour Doppler studies has led to great advances in the assessment of the heart and blood vessels, with flow being demonstrated with anatomical precision. Cardiac ultrasound allows assessment of the valves, as well as precise measurement of myocardial function. These techniques also allow vessel stenoses to be identified in areas such as the carotid bifurcation.

Most ultrasound studies are carried out in the abdominal organs, since good views of the liver, kidneys, pancreas and spleen can be obtained. The images produced show the anatomical form of the organ, allowing masses and dilatation to be seen, and the reflectivity of the tissues determines whether the areas appear bright (highly reflective) or dark (poor reflectors). Water reflects very poorly, as it has no internal boundaries to generate echoes. Fluid-filled structures such as the gallbladder or bladder are therefore shown as black voids. Individual organs have characteristic patterns of echo returns, depending on the distribution of fat (reflective) and other tissues within them.

Tumours and other mass lesions can have higher or lower echogenicity, or may be the same as the organ in which they lie. Cysts and other fluid-filled collections will be dark, but debris, blood, or pus within them can raise their echogenicity towards or above that of the surrounding tissues.

Stones reflect all the incident sound at their leading surface, and thus appear as a bright boundary with a comet-tail shadow behind where there is no 'illuminating' sound beam and thus no view (Fig. 1.2).

Check for:

Liver: metastases, abscess, biliary dilatation, enlargement/shrinkage in cirrhosis.

Gallbladder: stones, common duct stones.

Pancreas: tumours, pseudocysts.

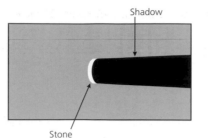

Figure 1.2 Acoustic shadow caused by stone on ultrasound.

Kidneys: size, scarring, masses, hydronephrosis, cysts, simple and polycystic kidney disease.

Spleen: size, masses.

Para-aortic region: lymph nodes.

Peritoneum: ascites, tumours, collections.

Computed tomography

This presents cross-sectional views of the body, which should always be viewed from the patient's feet looking upwards, so that the right side of the patient is the left side of the image (Fig. 1.3). The image is a map of the density of the tissues in the slice. Bone and areas of high density will be white. Low-density areas, such as air, are black. Soft tissues are close to the density of water, and usually appear as shades of grey.

It is possible to manipulate the image to show different areas of the same slice (windowing). This is necessary, as details in the lungs and the mediastinum require different settings to allow them to be seen well.

The injection of contrast medium will increase the density of vessels and tissue with a high vascular content. This can increase the visibility of lesions—making them more dense than normal tissue, or revealing them when the normal tissues enhance, exposing the lesion as a lower-density area.

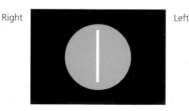

Figure 1.3 Patient orientation on a CT image.

New computer techniques allow sophisticated data manipulation, creating three-dimensional models of tumours and organs and allowing arteriograms to be generated without the need for intra-arterial catheter insertion.

Head

Look for symmetry, midline shift, areas of high or low density, and calcification. The ventricles can be enlarged by loss of cerebral substance as well as raised pressure. Tumours may only be seen after the injection of contrast material, or due to the surrounding low-density oedema. Gross oedema is classically seen in metastases.

The CT features of a cerebrovascular accident can take 24 hours or more to show. Blood can vary from high density (acute) to low density (chronic), depending on its age. Extradurals are lens-shaped, limited by the stripped dura, whereas subdurals conform to the cerebral surface. Subarachnoid blood is best seen as high-density areas in the cerebrospinal fluid recesses.

Check the pituitary region, the bones of the skull and the orbits for unexpected pathology.

Spine

The spinal CT can be with or without intrathecal contrast. Intrathecal contrast allows the presence of intradural and intraspinal abnormalities to be demonstrated.

The plain CT demonstrates lesions in or adjacent to the bone well. Look for extension of any mass lesion through the foramina.

Thorax

The thoracic CT can be directed at the lung, with high-resolution tomography (slice thickness of 1 mm or less) allowing detailed assessment of the parenchyma in interstitial diseases. Using thicker slices of 5–10 mm allows three-dimensional assessment of the lungs and mediastinum for tumour or other pathologies, such as bronchiectasis. Look at lungs for the pattern of parenchyma and for any areas of consolidation.

In the mediastinum, vessels will be better seen on contrast-enhanced scans. Lymph nodes should be looked for in their anatomical key sites: hilar, subcarinal, paratracheal.

The air spaces, both bronchial and parenchymal, should be checked for obstruction or masses. Remember that pus, mucus and fluid are all close to water and their density alone cannot separate them: it is the associated pattern of changes that will help discriminate between them.

As always, check the bones for occult pathology, e.g. metastases.

Abdomen

Check each organ individually, looking at each available slice it appears on. The chosen slices will contain the lesion or lesions; don't assume that because only part of an organ is seen, this is not the key area.

Check for:

Liver. Lesions can be higher or lower than the normal density. Cysts can be single or multiple, have smooth walls and are low in density. Check for dilated biliary radicals, and follow the bile duct through to the duodenum for stones or masses.

Spleen. Look for size and focal abnormalities. If it is enlarged, check for features of portal hypertension such as ascites and liver changes, or for nodal enlargement in lymphoma.

Pancreas. Tumour, pseudocyst, atrophy and calcification.

Kidneys. Size, shape, masses, calcification, dilatation.

Adrenal glands. These lie close to the upper pole of the kidneys. The right one is sometimes behind the interior vena cava.

Para-aortic region. Lymph nodes, aneurysmal dilatation of the aorta, abscess in the psoas muscle? Tuberculosis from the spine.

Bowel. Look for dilatation in obstruction or inflammation. Check for thickening of the wall or tumour masses.

Uterus and ovaries. Size, shape, masses, calcification.

Peritoneum. Ascites, abscess, tumour deposits.

Check the bones and abdominal wall for surprise lesions and for evidence of previous surgery that might point towards a diagnosis.

Magnetic resonance imaging

This technique differs significantly from CT—although the images superficially resemble CT images, the information they contain is profoundly different. The CT image shows tissue densities, whereas MRI depicts the signal strengths of the various tissues, which differ greatly depending on the image sequence used. CT uses large doses of radiation, but in MRI the technique has no known long-term hazards.

The commonest studies are T1-weighted and T2-weighted images. In T1 images, fat shows up as a high signal (white), water as a low signal (dark) and muscle as intermediate (grey). In T2 scans, water becomes the high signal (white), while fat becomes less bright and muscle also darkens. Oedema is therefore seen as an ill-defined fluid spread through an area of tissue. There are over 500 different MRI sequences now available, and a comprehensive description of the appearances seen for each organ and condition would be beyond the scope of this introduction.

MRI is excellent at imaging soft tissues, and allows unparalleled assessment of the brain, spinal cord and musculoskeletal system, including the bone marrow. Newer techniques, such as magnetic resonance angiography (MRA), also allow the heart, abdominal organs and vessels to be assessed non-invasively. The value of these techniques is rapidly approaching and, in certain cases has already overtaken, that of conventional modalities. The images are presented in a form that mimics conventional angiograms.

Tumour and infection are seen by their mass effects and associated local tissue oedema.

MRI has an additional benefit over CT in that the areas can be scanned in any plane—coronal, sagittal, or transverse—allowing excellent three-dimensional visualization of pathology. As in CT, the addition of intravenous contrast agents can highlight areas of increased vascularity or damaged blood–tissue boundaries.

Nuclear medicine

This often underestimated modality has great diagnostic power, since it demonstrates the metabolic functioning of the organs that are imaged, whereas the majority of imaging techniques show only the morphological patterns. The process relies on the injection of selected tracer molecules that target—i.e. are selectively taken up by—specific organs. These are 'labelled' by a radioactive tracer atom (commonly technetium), which by emitting gamma photons allows the site of the molecules' uptake to be imaged.

The key step in interpreting an isotope study is to recognize the organ imaged. This will guide you in identifying the study type and thus the potential pathologies to be seen.

All studies are maps of the distribution of the isotope, and identifying areas in which the activity is either higher or lower than normal is therefore one of the key features of interpretation. High activity indicates greater than normal function, and low activity shows reduced or absent function. It is important to remember that a finite amount of isotope is injected in each study. In extreme cases, therefore, almost all the activity can be concentrated in one area, leaving the surrounding 'normal' areas looking reduced in activity. This is best seen in bone scans, in which the normal situation shows excretion of isotope into the renal tract, with the kidneys appearing. However, in the 'superscan' that occurs in diffuse disseminated metastases, all activity is locked into the bone, with no focally high activity. The absence of activity in the kidneys acts as a marker for the condition.

Ventilation–perfusion scan

The study most often performed is the ventilation–perfusion (V/Q) scan. This can be identified by the matched pairs of images. One shows the spread of inhaled isotope (often krypton) demonstrating the ventilated areas of lung, and the other is the perfusion map of the distribution of an injected macromolecule tagged with technetium, which lodges in the pulmonary capillary bed. Mismatch segments can show evidence of pulmonary emboli, with holes in the perfusion that do not match with ventilation defects. Matched defects occur in diffuse pulmonary diseases such as asthma and chronic obstructive airway disease (COAD).

Bone

Bone scanning demonstrates osteoblast activity, i.e. bone deposition. Hot spots occur in infection, tumour fractures and arthritis. Not all tumours elicit bone deposition. Classically, myeloma shows very poorly on bone scans, and skeletal surveys are therefore still necessary to identify lytic foci in this condition. Very large deposits may thus appear as cold spots, as can dead bone in avascular necrosis.

Kidney

The mainstays of the renography technique are:

1 Dimercaptosuccinic acid (DMSA), which is fixed in the tubule and demonstrates functioning renal parenchyma. Renal scars and cysts appear as cold areas in the kidney.

2 A dynamic study, either diethylenetriaminepentaacetic acid (DTPA) or mercaptoacetyltriglycine (MAG3).

These tracers are excreted into the urine, and dynamic scanning can thus demonstrate hold-ups in urine drainage, with the curve from one kidney remaining high rather than falling exponentially as the tracer is eluted from the kidney by fresh urine. The technique can also demonstrate renal artery stenosis; in this case, the peak activity in the affected kidney is lower and delayed in comparison with the contralateral kidney (beware of bilateral disease).

Both techniques have a role in identifying ectopic or atrophic renal tissue. In the transplanted kidney, they can also identify graft infarction. These studies are capable of replication to a high standard, and therefore allow function to be quantified and compared at different times.

Heart

Cardiac nuclear studies primarily focus on cardiac muscle perfusion. Cold areas may represent infarcts, aneurysms, or areas of ischaemia. The latter will fill on the resting-phase study. Such images are usually thallium studies, presented as horseshoe-shaped activity plots, in which the central ventricular cavity corresponds to the central zone of low activity.

Liver

Liver scanning is now essentially out of date, and has been replaced by ultrasound, CT and MRI. However, biliary studies are still occasionally performed.

Thyroid

The thyroid gland is seen as a bilobar structure with a marker for the sternal notch. Cold areas represent cysts, inactive nodules, or carcinomas. Retrosternal extension will be indicated by the marker. Parathyroid glands can be demonstrated by combined thallium-201 scans of the thyroid and parathyroid, with subtraction of a second thyroid-specific technetium study revealing the parathyroid tissue.

Adrenal glands

Adrenal scans for steroid and adrenaline-secreting tumours are available to localize the tumour, although CT is now the first-line imaging investigation.

Haematology

Red cell scanning for occult blood loss shows abnormal pooling of activity in segments of bowel. Indium-labelled white cell studies show very hazy concentrations of activity in inflammatory foci and abscess. Areas of inflammatory bowel disease can thus mimic or hide associated abscess formation in the abdomen.

Conclusion

This introduction is by necessity a rapid, highly selective discussion of the imaging modalities available to you in your clinical work (and thus also to the examiners). It cannot hope to cover every aspect of the role of imaging, particularly the ways in which disease manifests itself in the images produced. There is no substitute for experience in seeing images in order to connect their appearances with the pathologies encountered—particularly looking at the images of classical presentations that accompany the discussions of each disease in all standard medical texts.

Questions

Cardiology

1

A 29-year-old woman presents with a two-month history of shortness of breath after a miscarriage. She has had a pulmonary embolism during a previous pregnancy, and her only other past medical history is of epilepsy in her late teens and two previous miscarriages. Her ECG shows a sinus tachycardia with RBBB morphology.

What does her CXR show?
What is the diagnosis?
What is the likely aetiology of her condition?

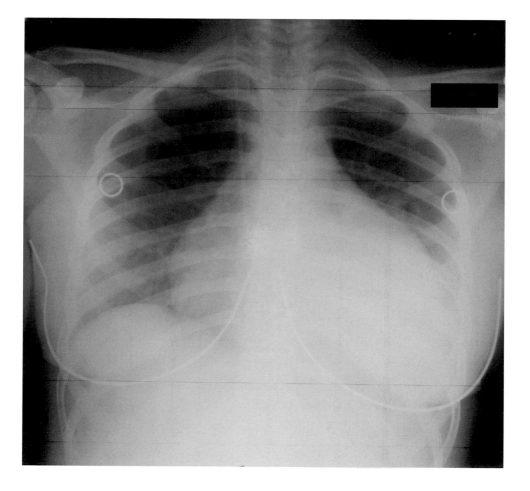

2   A 42-year-old woman complains of increasing tiredness, lethargy and intermittent haemoptysis. She is admitted for further investigations, and the following test is done (*see below and opposite*).

What is the test and what does it show?
What is the diagnosis?

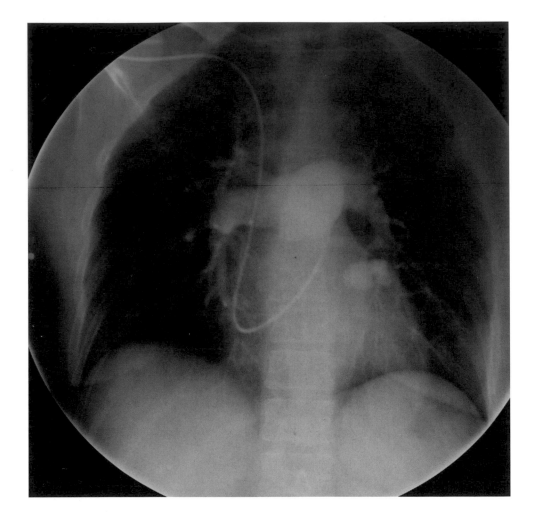

2

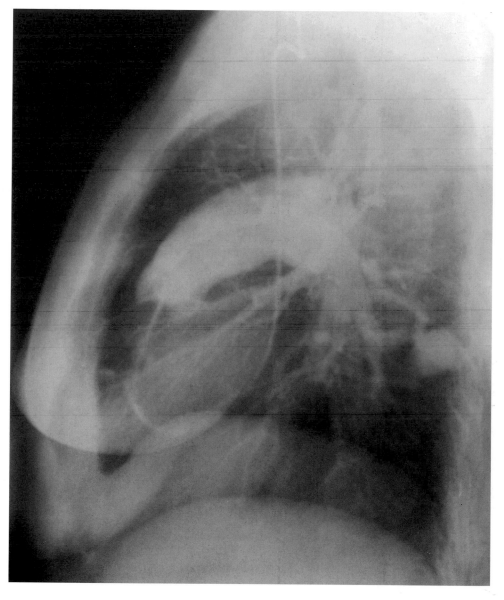

3

An 18-year-old army recruit is admitted to hospital with an episode of sharp pleuritic chest pain. His past medical history is unremarkable apart from frontal headaches. This is his CXR.

What does it show?
What is the diagnosis?
What is the probability of a male offspring having the same condition?

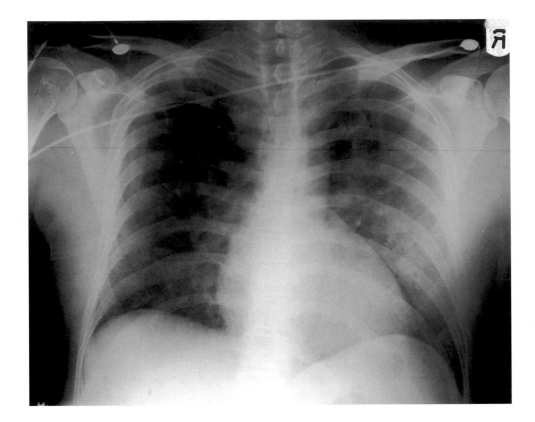

4

A 28-year-old man is referred to the outpatient department for investigation of a heart murmur. On direct questioning, he admits to increasing breathlessness on exertion. There is also a family history of heart murmurs, with one sibling dying suddenly when 30 years old. On examination, he has a late systolic murmur at the apex, radiating to the axilla. While awaiting further investigations, he is admitted to hospital with an episode of severe chest pain and breathlessness.

What does the following test show?
Which signs would you expect to find on auscultation of the heart?
What is the diagnosis?

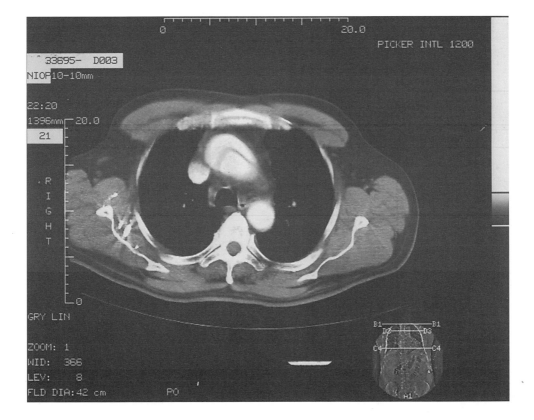

5

A 24-year-old man describes intermittent visual loss and blurring of vision. He sees his general practitioner, who finds no abnormality apart from quite marked hypertension. He is then sent for an ECG, which shows LVH, and a CXR, which is shown below.

What does it show?
What is the diagnosis?
What is the cause of the blurred vision?

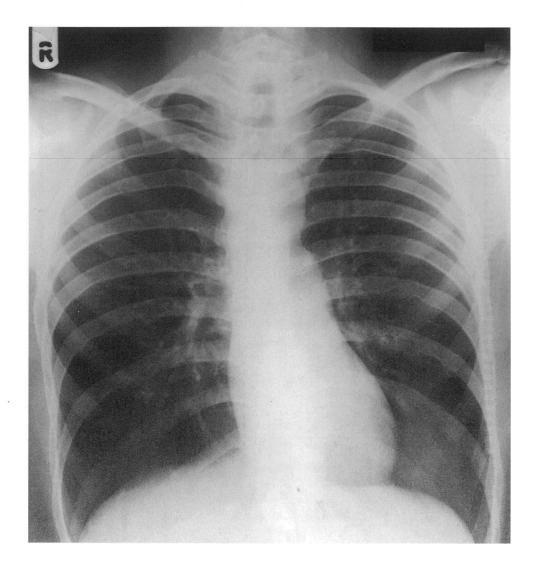

6   This is a CXR of a 30-year-old man with shortness of breath.

What does it show?
What is the diagnosis?

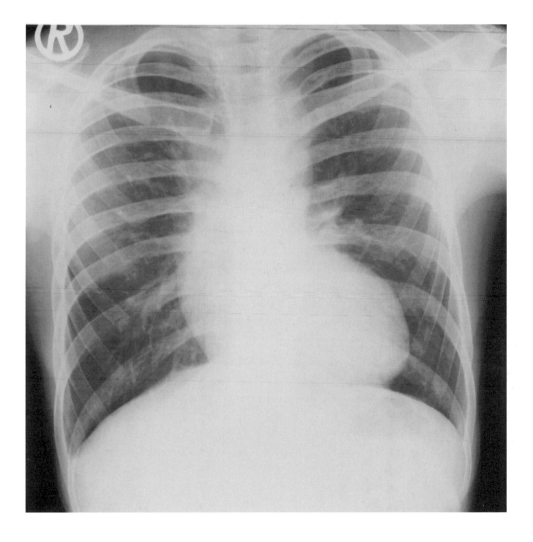

7   A 28-year-old woman is admitted to hospital with a stroke three days after leaving hospital following the birth of her child. Here is her CXR.

What does it show?
What is the diagnosis?
Which is the likely cause of her stroke?

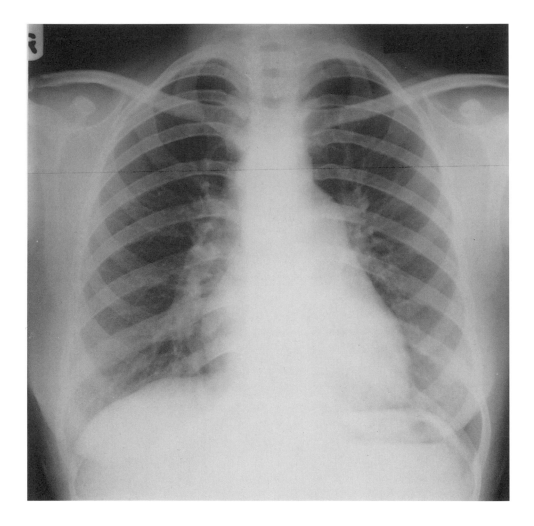

8 This is a CXR of a 38-year-old woman with progressive breathlessness (*see below and overleaf*).

What does it show?
What is the cause of her breathlessness?
How could you confirm the diagnosis?
Which signs might you find?

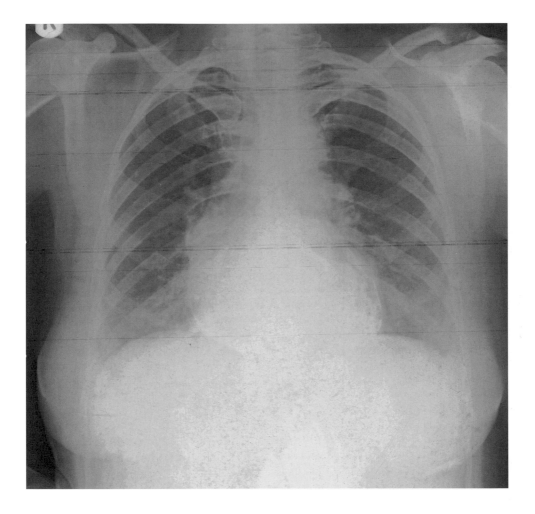

8

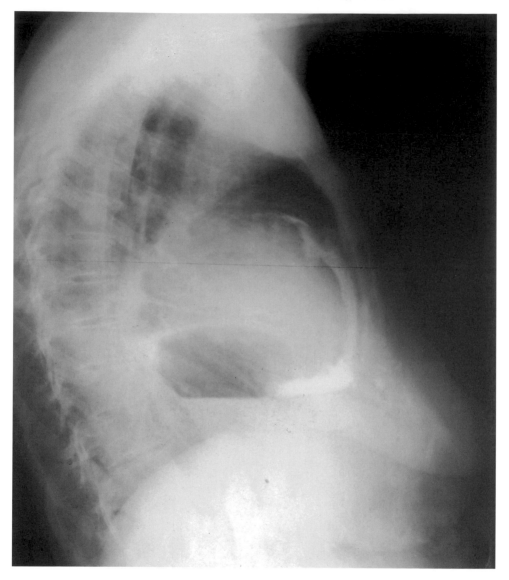

9   This is a CXR of a 68-year-old man with haemoptysis and shortness of breath.

What does it show?
What is the cause of the radiological abnormalities?
What is the cause of the haemoptysis?

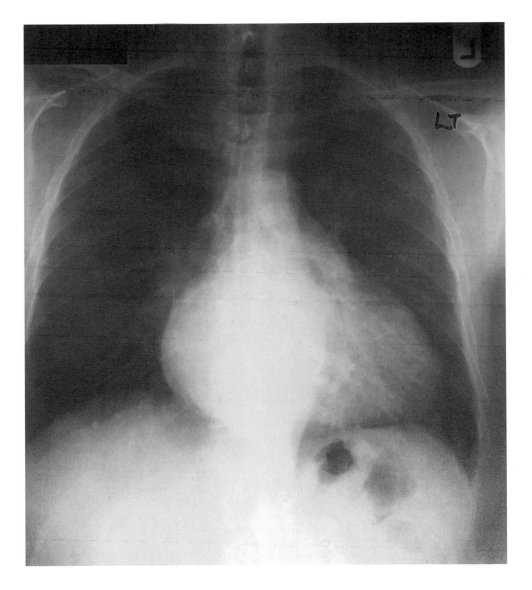

10
A young woman develops intermittent pain and numbness in her hands and feet. She also complains of a fever. Following exhaustive tests, an MRI scan of the thorax is done.

What does it show?
What is the diagnosis?

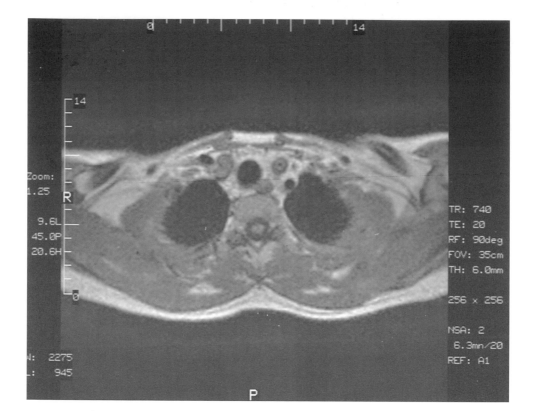

11

A 50-year-old man develops post-infarction angina. Since his infarction, he has had several TIAs. He undergoes cardiac catheterization following a positive exercise test. His LV angiogram is shown.

What does it show?
What is the cause of the TIAs?

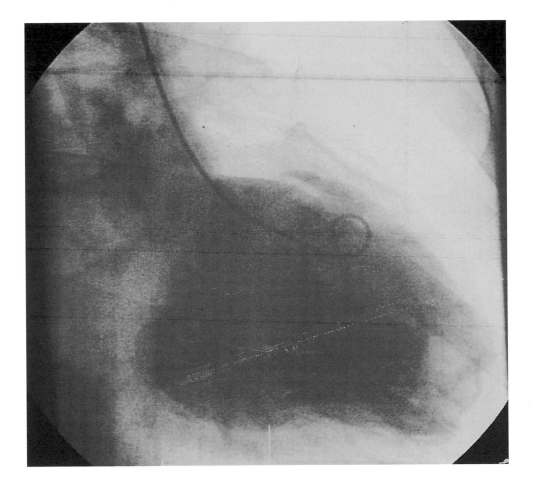

12   A 50-year-old woman complains of increasing dyspnoea on exertion. Here is her CXR.

What does it show?
Which procedure has she undergone in the past?

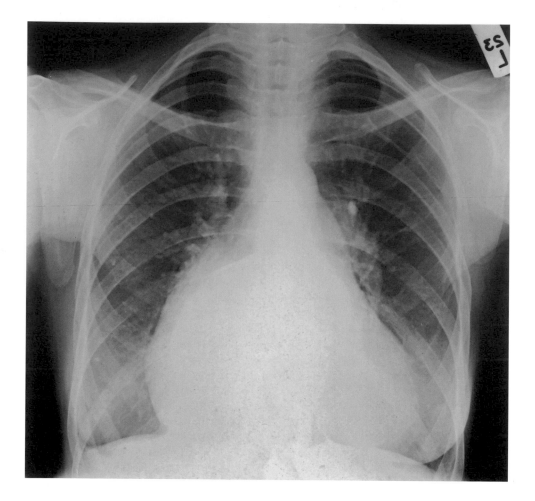

13
An 80-year-old man complains of backache that has persisted for six months. On further questioning, he admits to hesitancy and a poor stream. This is an X-ray of his lumbar spine.

What does it show?
What is the diagnosis?

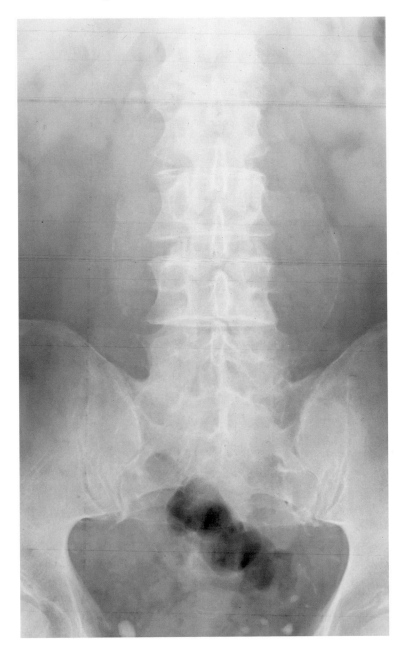

14

A 34-year-old man with hyperlipidaemia complains of shortness of breath on exertion. He has the test shown opposite (*see facing plate*) done.

Which test is this?
What does it show?
What would you do next?

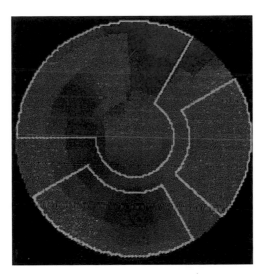

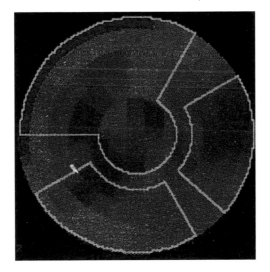

1

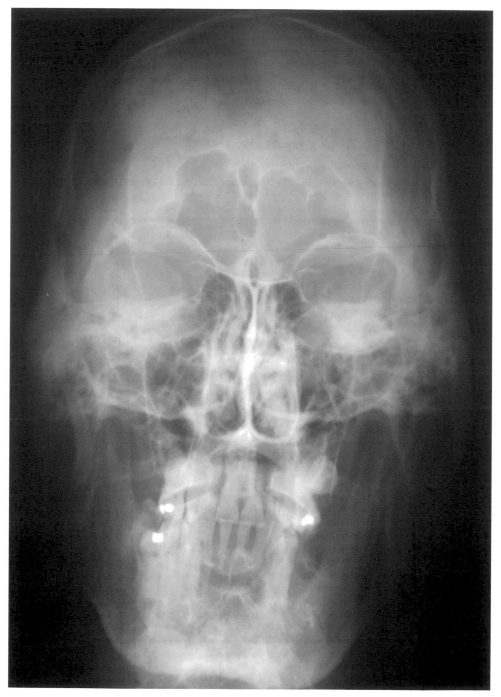

2

This is a radiograph of a man's hand.

What does it show?
What is the diagnosis?

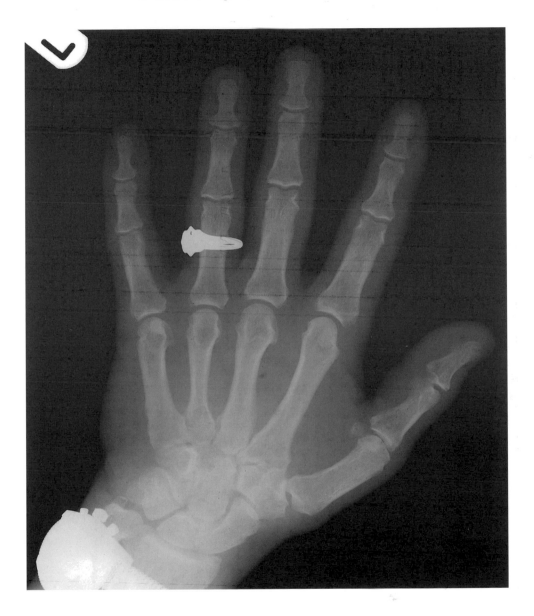

3   A man complains of general joint pain and tingling in his hands. This is an X-ray of his thoracolumbar spine.

Describe the abnormalities.
Name the condition that led to this appearance.

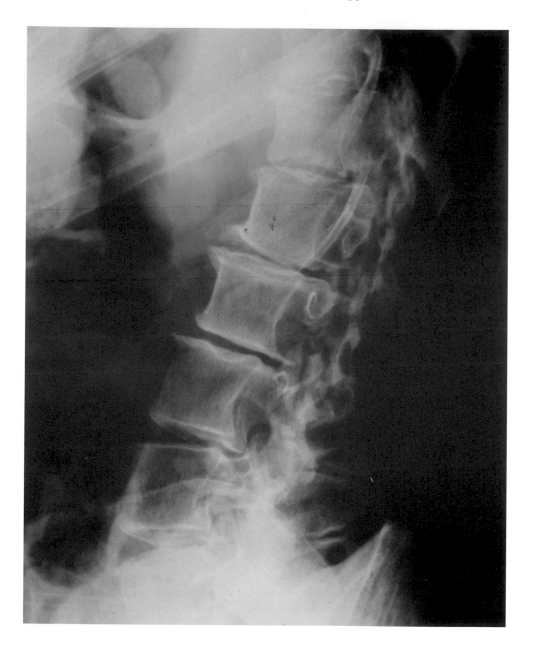

4   This is a CT scan of a 40-year-old man with diabetes (*see below and overleaf*). He presented with poor diabetic control. On direct questioning, he complained of headaches and excess sweating. Examination revealed a dorsal kyphosis, pes cavus and a pedunculated lesion on the tongue.

What does the CT show?
What is the diagnosis?
Which biochemical tests are mandatory?

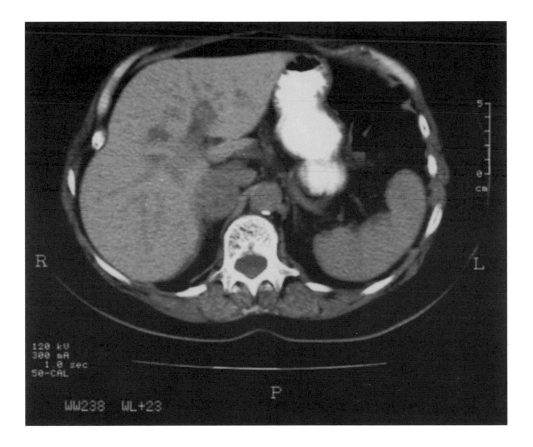

4

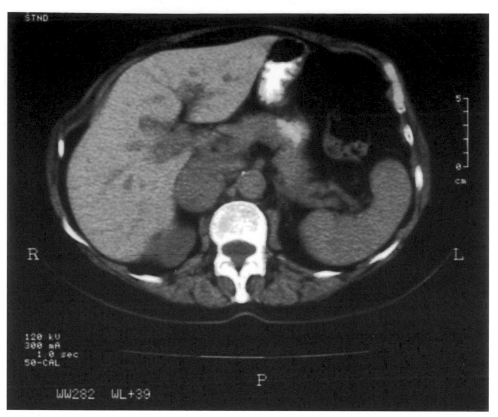

5

A 24-year-old woman presents with weight loss, vomiting, diarrhoea and episodes of dizziness. She loses consciousness in the admissions unit. On examination, she is a thin woman with a blood pressure of 90/60. Her capillary blood glucose is 1.8 mmol/L.

What does her X-ray show?
What is the cause of her presentation?
What might an abdominal X-ray show?

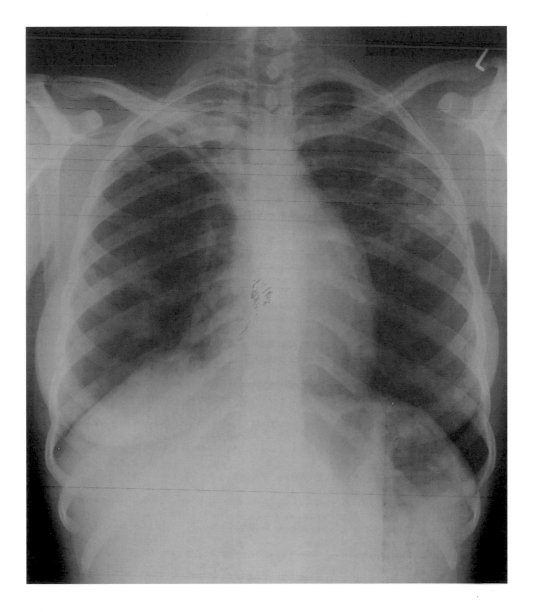

6   A 26-year-old woman under investigation for galactorrhoea complains of diplopia. On examination, she has a sixth nerve palsy. An MRI scan of the head is shown.

What does it show?
What is the diagnosis?
What is the cause of the sixth nerve palsy?

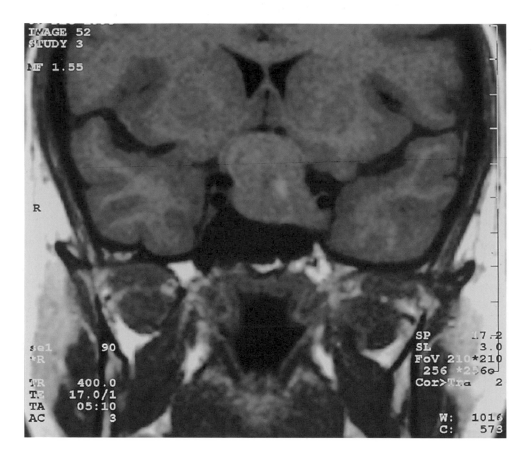

7   A 46-year-old woman, in psychiatric care for a personality disorder, complains of malaise, vomiting and abdominal pain. A dipstick of her urine shows haematuria. These are X-rays of her skull and hands (*see below and overleaf*).

What do they show?
What is the diagnosis?
What is the cause of the haematuria?

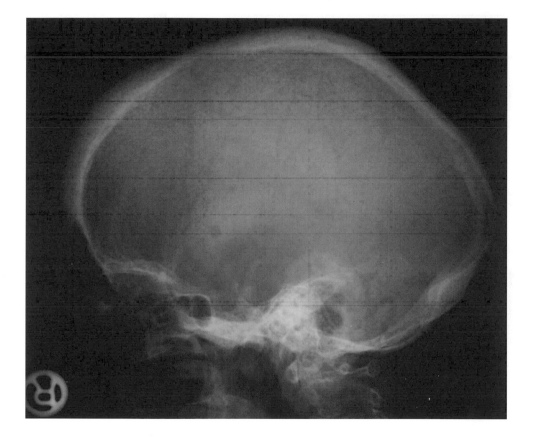

7

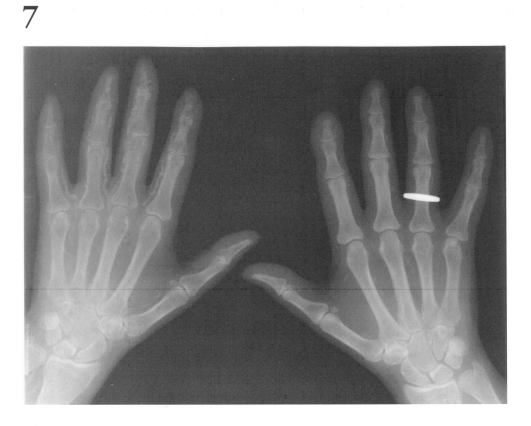

8   This is an X-ray of the hands of a 20-year-old man with a learning disability.

What does it show?
What is the diagnosis?

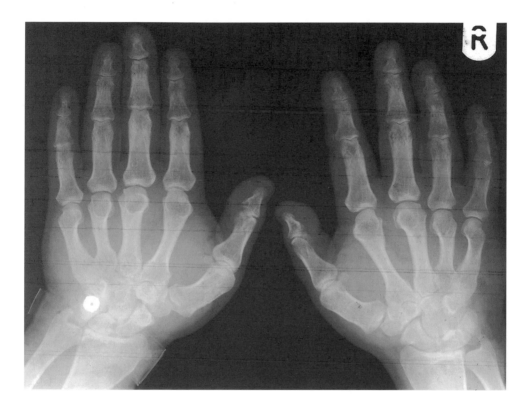

9

A 60-year-old woman presented with left heart failure. On examination, she was cachectic, with signs of overt pulmonary oedema. Her heart failure responds to conventional medical therapy.

Which investigation is shown?
What is the diagnosis?
Which eye signs might be present?

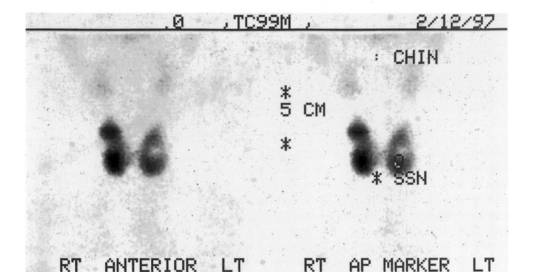

10   A 50-year-old woman presented with malaise, nausea and vomiting. She complained of headaches and bumping into objects. Serum biochemistry revealed hyponatraemia. This is an MRI scan (*see below*).

Why is she bumping into objects?
What is the diagnosis?

The patient underwent surgery. This is an X-ray two months later (*see overleaf*). Which complication has occurred?

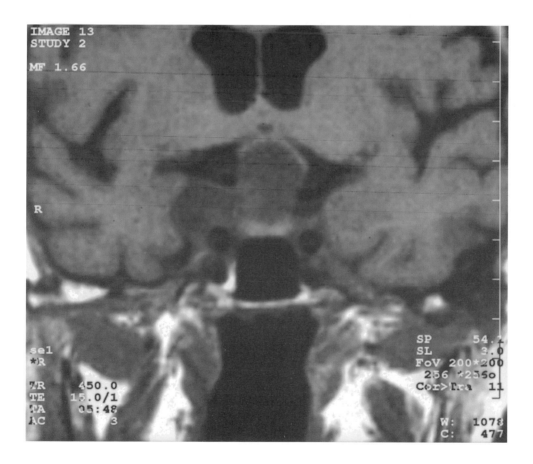

10

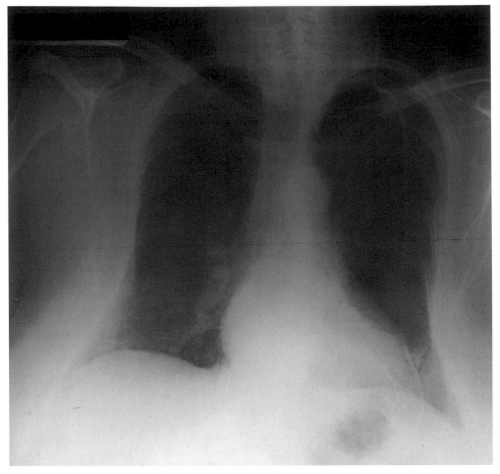

11 A 60-year-old woman complains of fullness in the neck and difficulty swallowing. These are her X-rays (*see below and overleaf*).

What do they show?
Which test would you do?
What is the diagnosis?

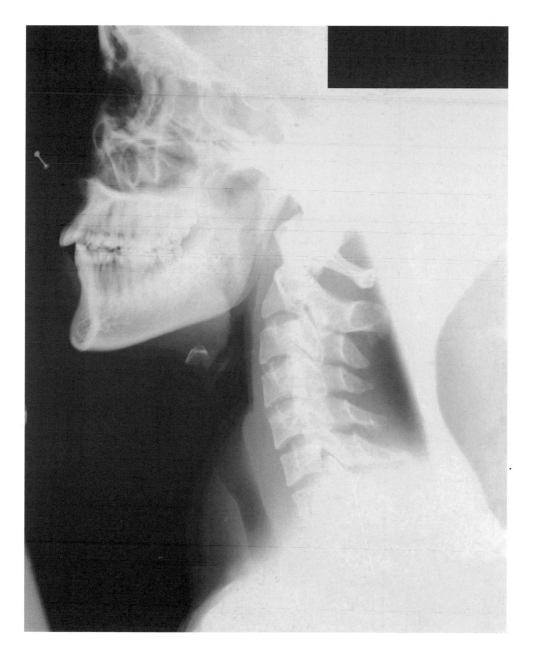

11

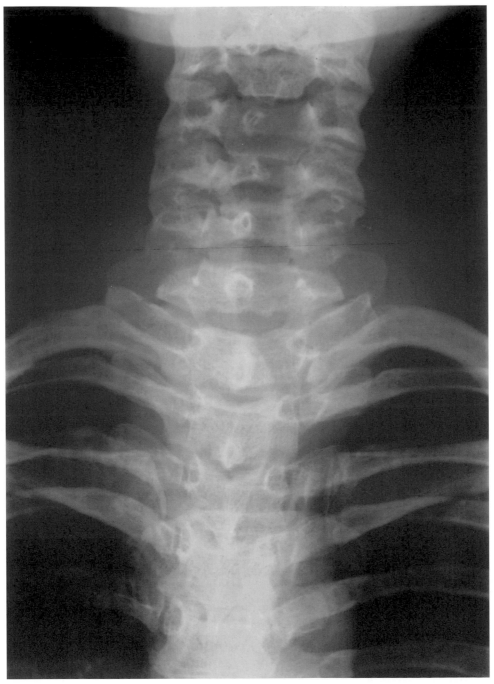

12   A 50-year-old woman presents with confusion and renal failure.

What is the scan?
What do the scans show?
What is the cause of the renal failure?

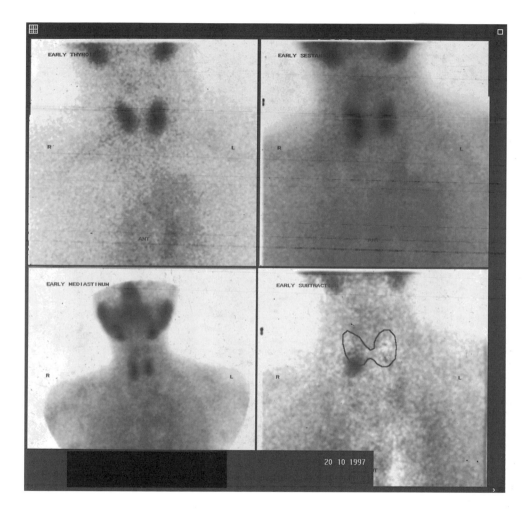

13   This is a radiograph of a 70-year-old Asian woman with weight loss.

What does the radiograph show?
What is the diagnosis?
What would you do next?

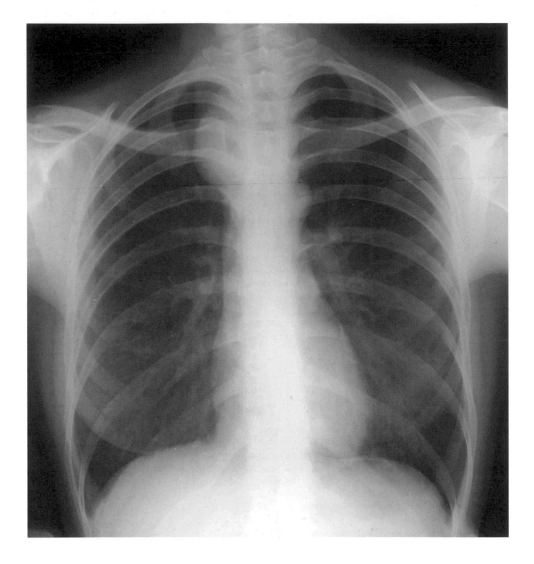

Gastroenterology

1

A 38-year-old man complains of dysphagia of eight months' duration. A full blood count shows a hypochromic microcytic anaemia. This is his barium swallow (*see below and overleaf*).

What does it show?
What is the diagnosis?

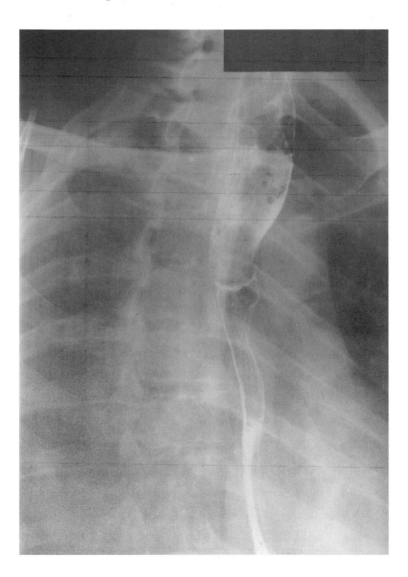

1

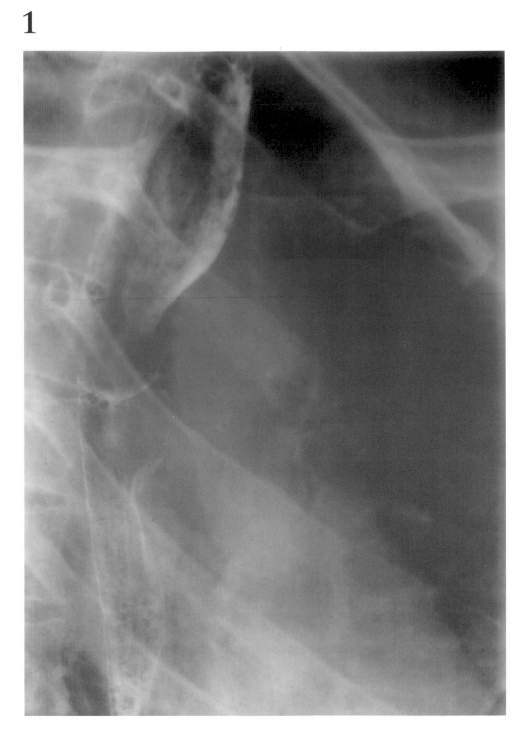

2

A 22-year-old man develops colicky abdominal pain. On examination, he is distressed and has marked pigmentation around his lips and hands. His abdomen is distended, with marked tenderness and reduced bowel sounds.

What does the X-ray investigation (*see below*) show?
What does the barium study (*see overleaf*) demonstrate?
What is the diagnosis?
Name two other complications of this condition.

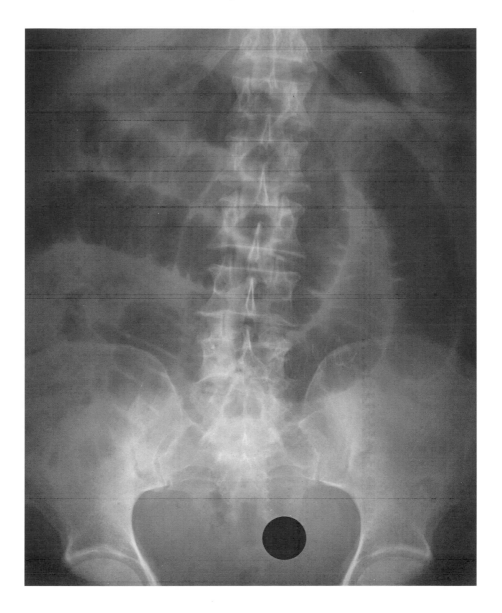

2

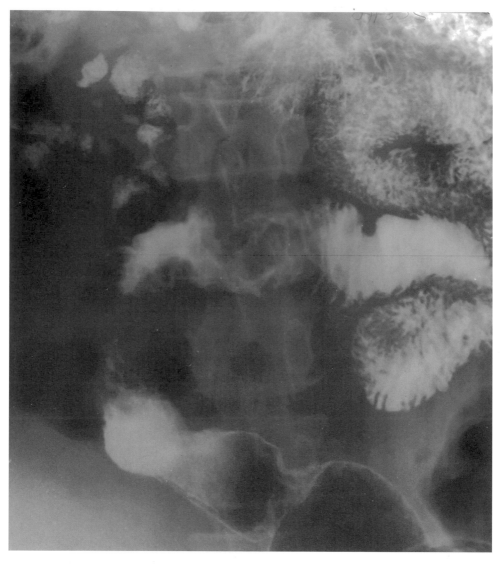

3 A 38-year-old man presents with a six-month history of passing dark urine. He has a past medical history of inflammatory bowel disease. His serum biochemistry shows a bilirubin of 80 μmol/L, AST of 210 IU/L, ALT 340 IU/L, and an alkaline phosphatase of 860 IU/L.

What does the following study show?
What is the diagnosis?
Which other complications may occur?

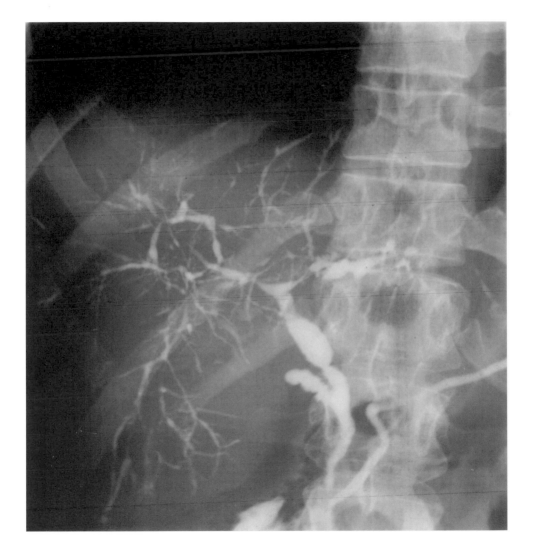

4   A 16-year-old girl is referred to hospital for investigation of her short stature. She has had intermittent episodes of abdominal pain and diarrhoea over the previous two years, which have settled. Her Hb is 9.8 g/dL with an MCV of 106 fl. These are barium studies of the girl done 1 year apart (*see below and opposite*).

What do they show?
What is the cause of her anaemia?

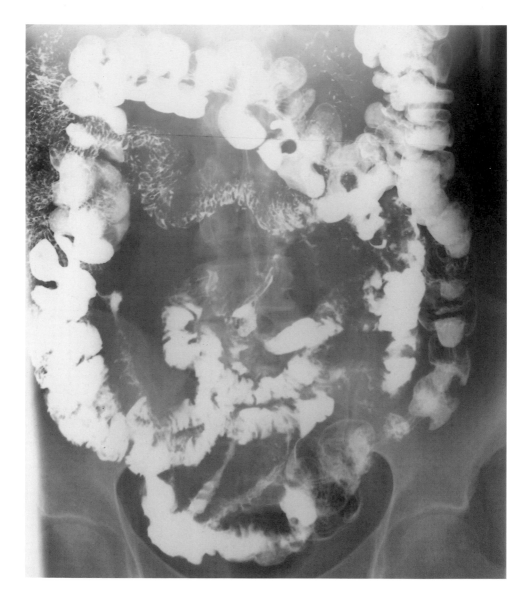

4

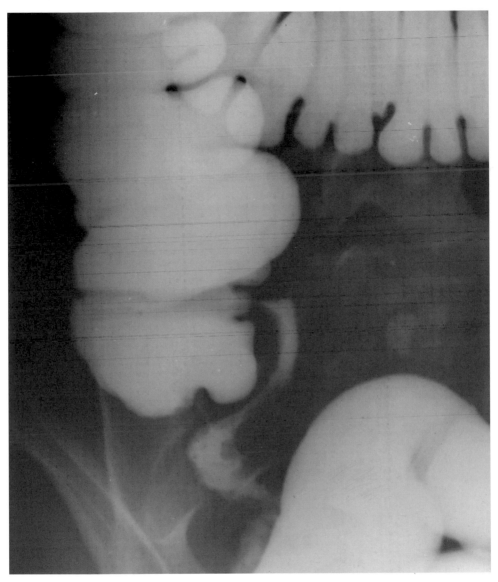

5   This is a CXR of a 64-year-old woman with shortness of breath and chest pain. On examination, she is pyrexial with a temperature of 37.6 °C, and has coarse crepitations at the right lung base. During the previous year, she has had recurrent episodes of chest pain associated with SOB and fever. On each occasion, the condition has responded to a course of broad-spectrum antibiotics. This is the CXR.

What does it show?
What is the cause of the recurrent chest infections?

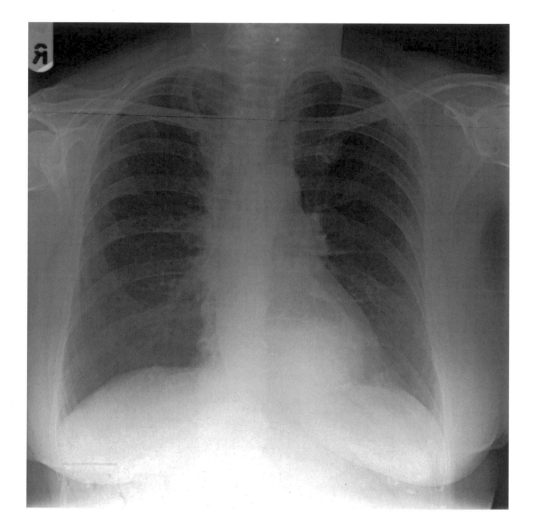

6 A 60-year-old woman is referred to the outpatient department for investigation of weight loss. This is her barium study.

What does it show?
What is the diagnosis?
Which complications can occur?

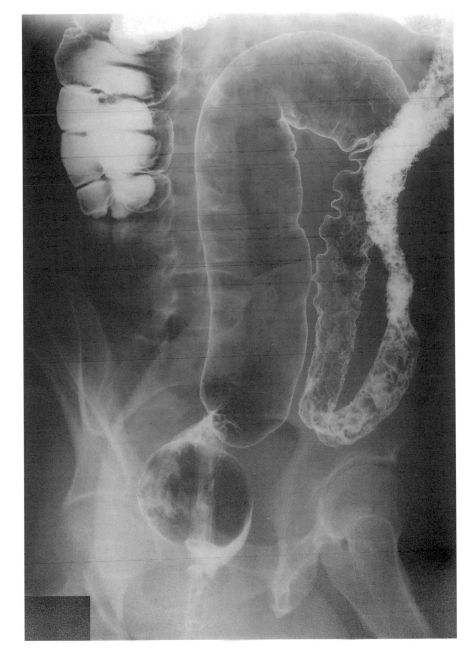

7   A 64-year-old man develops diabetes mellitus. He has a poor response to oral hypoglycaemic agents, and requires insulin. Despite careful dietary monitoring and dose adjustment, he complains of episodes of dizziness and sweating. The serum glucose measurement during one such attack is 2 mmol/L. He is subsequently admitted with abdominal pain and passing frequent pale stools. This is his AXR.

What does it show?
What is the aetiology of his diabetes?
Give two possible reasons for his hypoglycaemia.

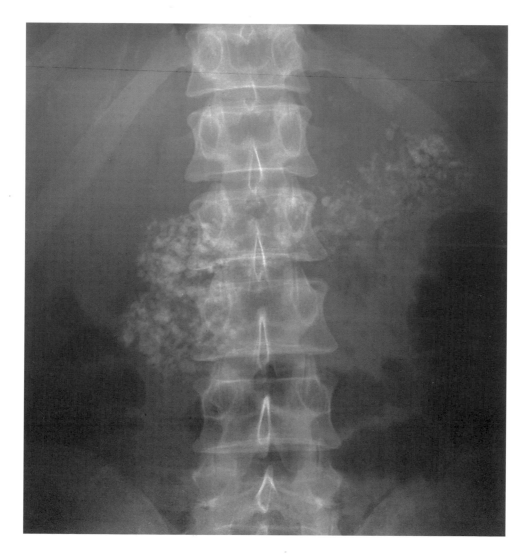

8   A 74-year-old woman complains of anorexia and weight loss that
have continued for six months. Her liver enzymes are as follows:
alkaline phosphatase 1000 IU/L, AST 136 IU/L, ALT 189 IU/L
and bilirubin 80 μmol/L.

What does the ERCP show (*see below and overleaf*)?
What is the likely differential diagnosis?

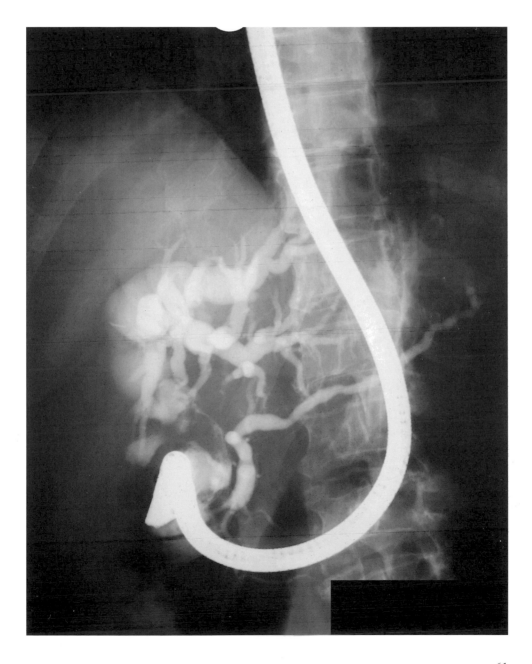

8

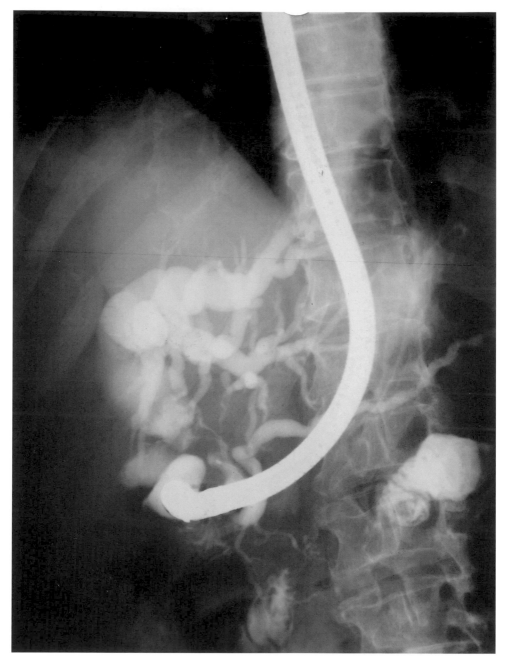

9

A 76-year-old woman develops colicky abdominal pain and is passing dark urine. An ultrasound scan is carried out, which is normal. Her symptoms settle, and she remains well. Six months later, the symptoms recur. A US scan is carried out, which shows a dilated biliary tree but no gallstones. An ERCP is carried out, which is shown below.

What does it show?
What is the cause of the abdominal pain?

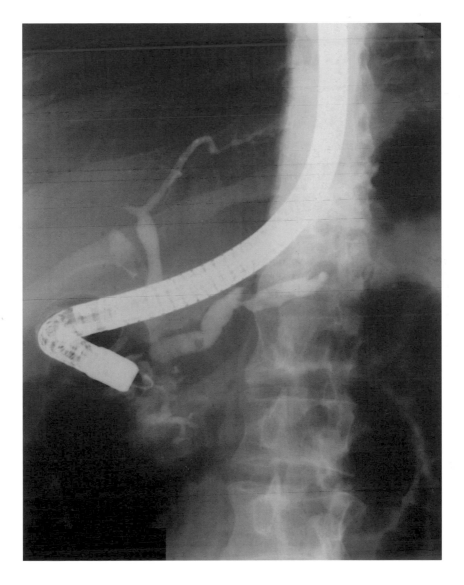

10
A businessman develops jaundice after a trip to the Far East. On direct questioning, he describes a similar episode after a trip to Hong Kong, which was attributed to a virus. He is a non-smoker and takes only modest amounts of alcohol. There is no history of IV drug use. He has had unprotected intercourse on previous trips abroad. On examination, he is icteric with 4 cm hepatomegaly. This is a CT scan of the abdomen.

What does it show?
What is the diagnosis?
What is the likely aetiology of the condition?

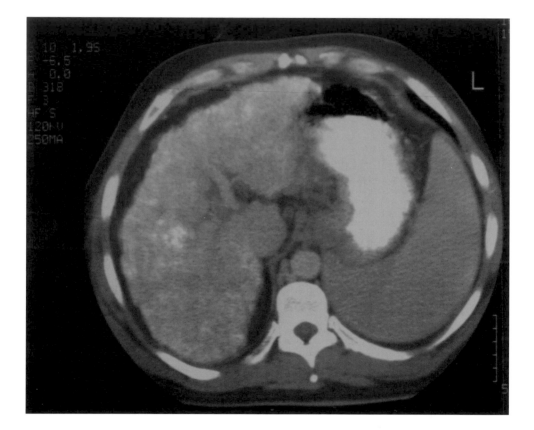

11   A 65-year-old man with a history of gallstones develops a swinging fever and rigors. Routine biochemistry shows markedly deranged LFTs. This is a CT scan of his abdomen.

What does it show?
What is the diagnosis?

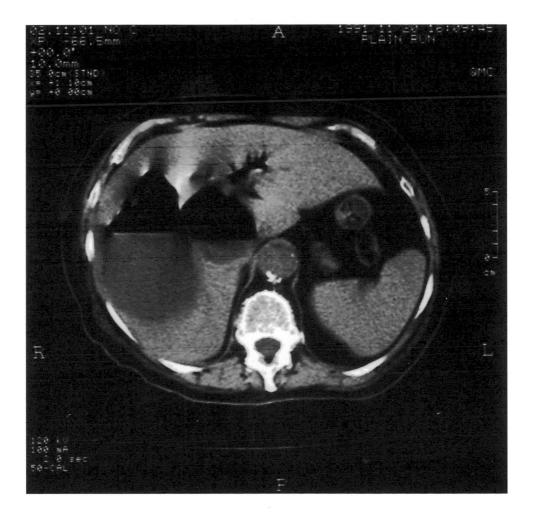

12   This is a barium study of a 45-year-old man.

What does it show?
What is the diagnosis?
What is this condition associated with?

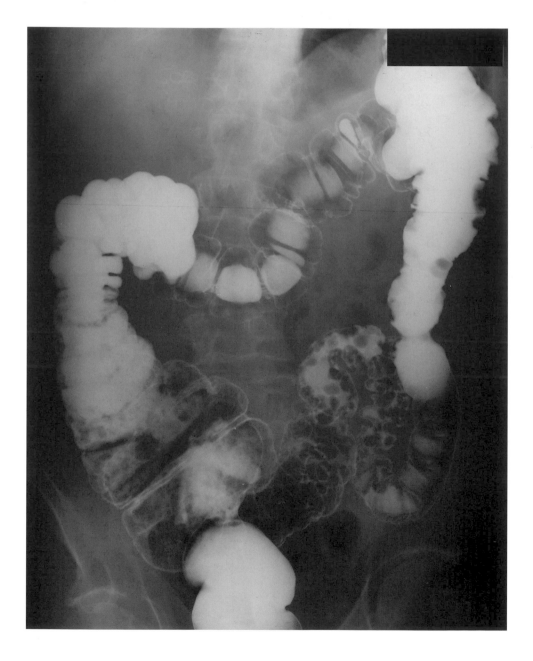

13   This is a barium study of a young man with a long history of rectal bleeding (*see below and overleaf*).

What does it show?

These are intravenous urograms and skull X-rays of the same man (*see pp. 69 & 70*).

What is the diagnosis?

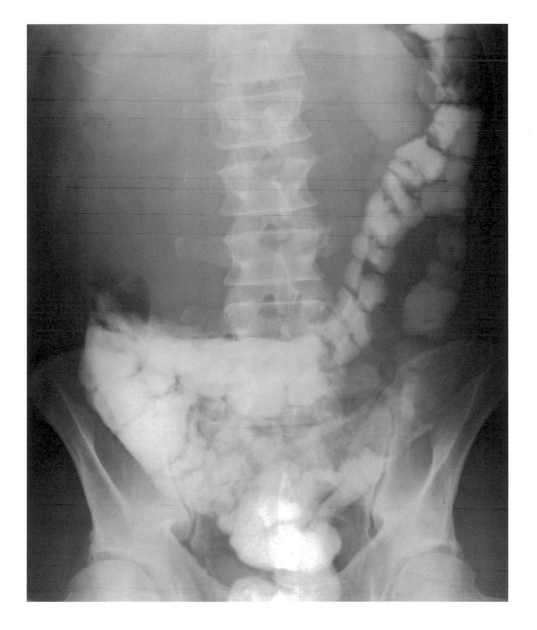

13

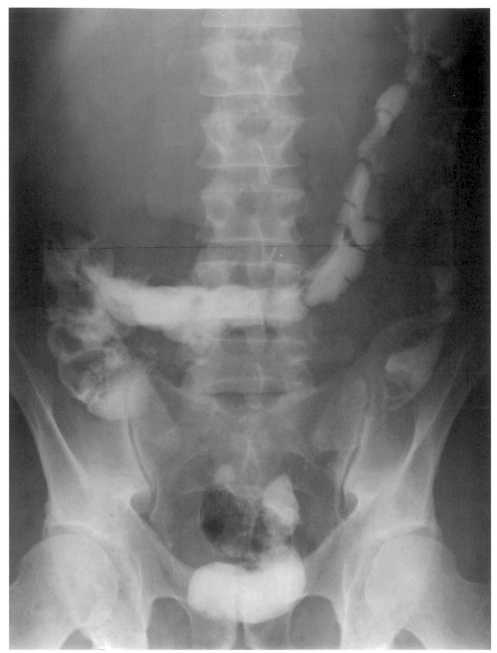

13

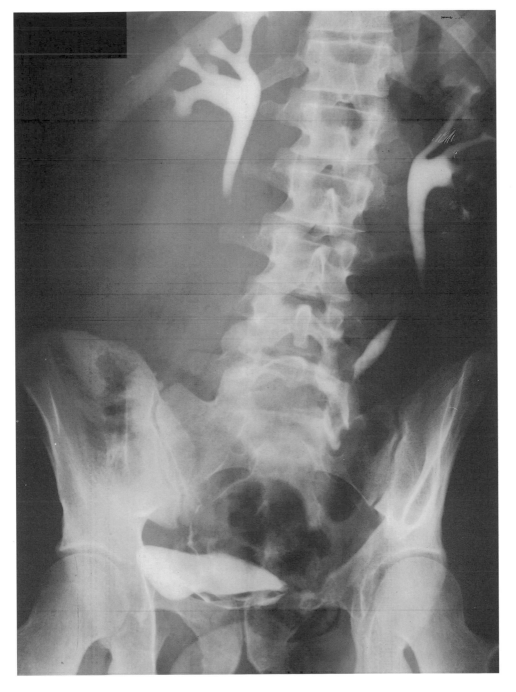

13

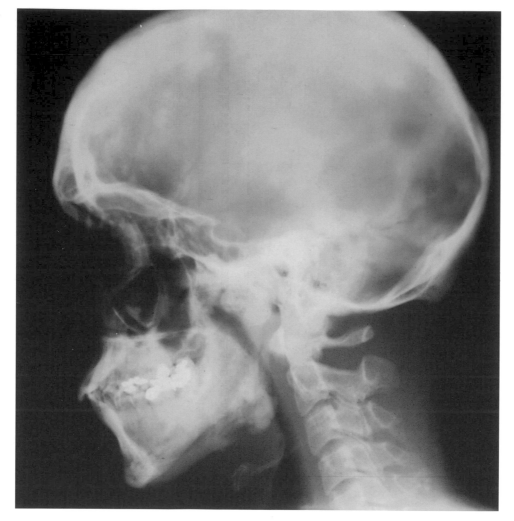

14 This is a barium swallow study in a 60-year-old man with dyspepsia.

What does it show?
What is the diagnosis?

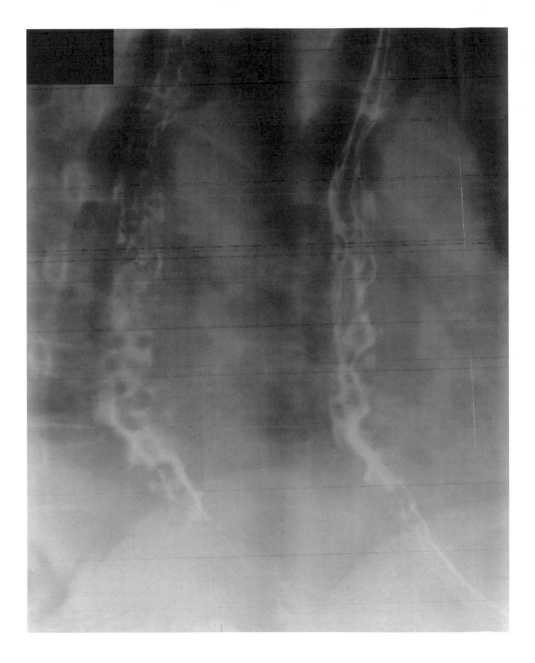

15
A 40-year-old heroin addict complains of a two-week history of odynophagia. On further questioning, he has a one-year history of weight loss and recurrent chest infections. This is his barium swallow.

What is the likely diagnosis?
What is the likely aetiology?
What is the differential diagnosis?

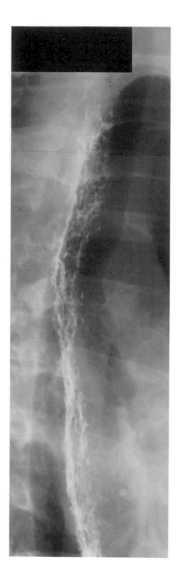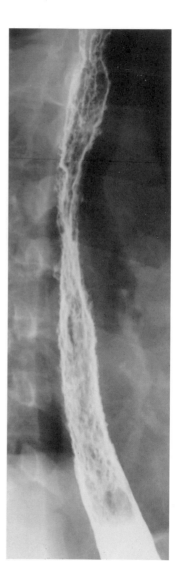

16

A 61-year-old woman complains of difficulty with swallowing and vomiting. During the previous year, she has had three hospital admissions with pneumonia. This is a barium swallow (*see below and overleaf*).

What does it show?
What is the diagnosis?

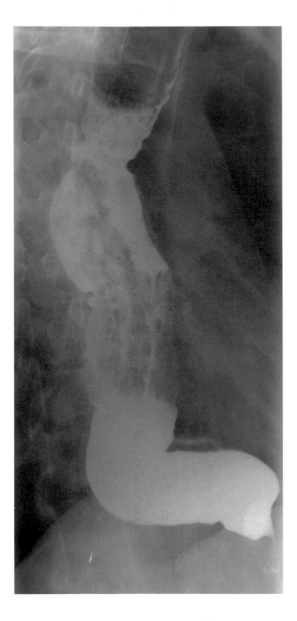

16

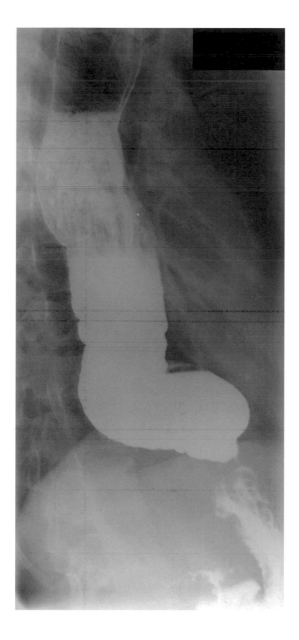

17   This is a barium meal study in a 40-year-old man with abdominal pain.

What does it show?
What would you do next?

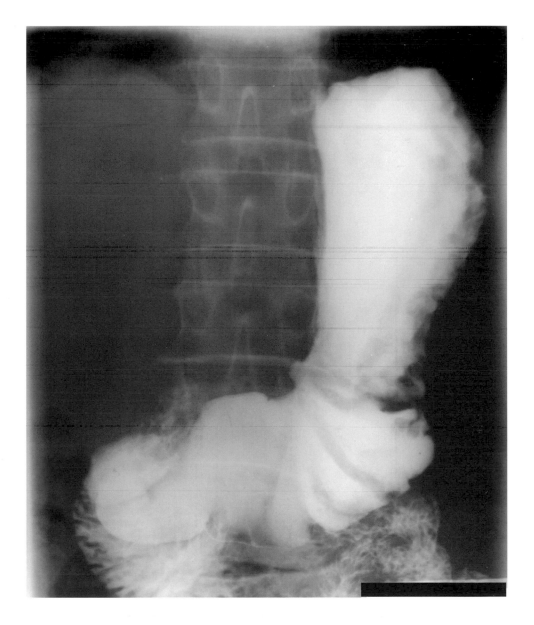

18 This is a barium meal study in a 60-year-old woman with abdominal pain (*see below and opposite*). One year later, she presents with a sudden onset of abdominal pain and vomiting. On examination, she is hypotensive and grey, with a rigid abdomen. Her WCC was 14×10^9/L; her urea and electrolytes were normal, but her Ca was elevated, with low PO_4. A plain X-ray is shown on p. 78. Her PMH includes treatment for a prolactinoma, and she is currently taking bromocriptine and ranitidine only.

What do the X-rays show?
What is the cause?
What is the aetiology of the radiological appearance, and which test would you do to confirm it?
Give a possible unifying diagnosis of this woman's condition.

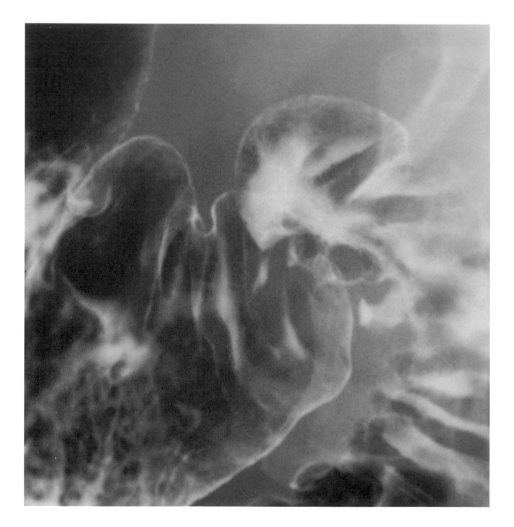

18

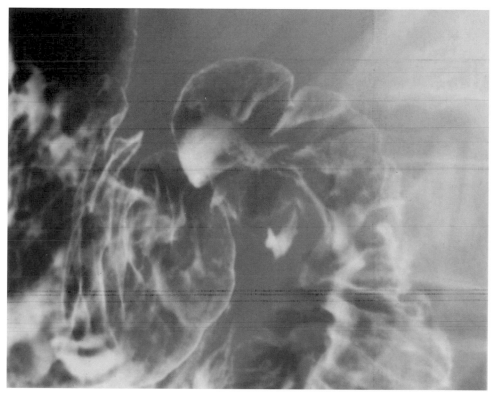

18

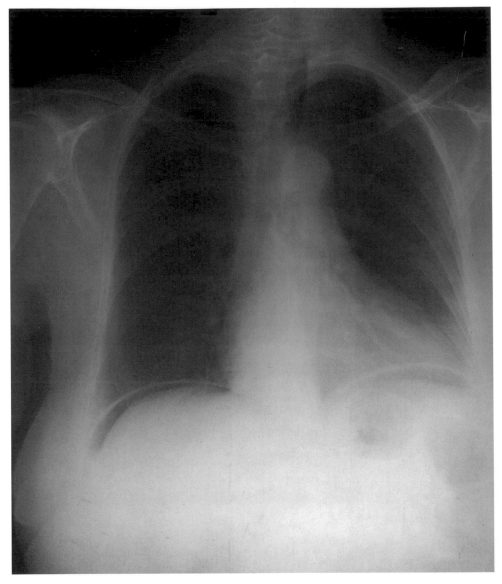

19 A 65-year-old woman with systemic sclerosis complains of weight loss, diarrhoea and lethargy. On examination, she is pale and has bilateral pitting oedema and weakness of her proximal muscles. Her Hb is 8 g/dL with an MCV of 104 fl. This is her barium follow-through.

What does it show?
What is the diagnosis?
What is the cause of her anaemia?
What is the cause of her muscle weakness?
Give the aetiology of her various symptoms. Which test would you do to confirm the diagnosis?

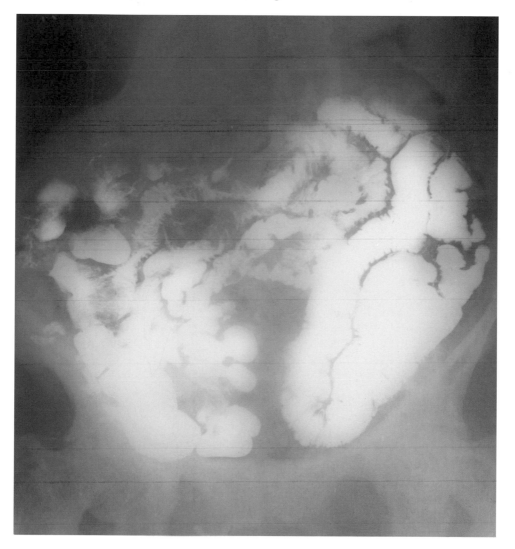

20   A 16-year-old Asian boy complains of colicky abdominal pain and loss of appetite. This is a barium study.

What is the diagnosis?
Which other symptoms might he have, and which tests would you do?

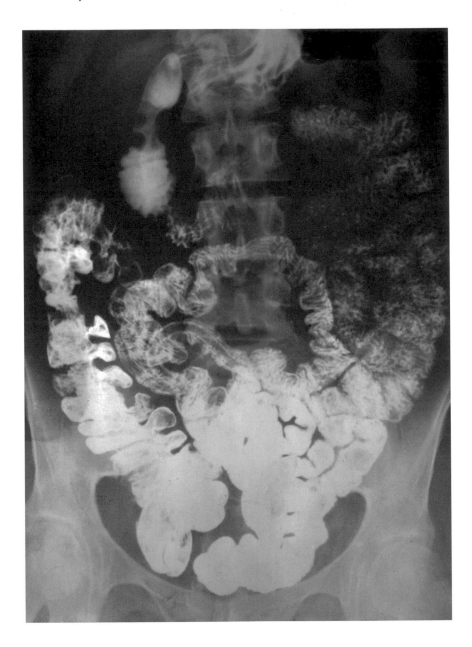

21   An 80-year-old woman presents with severe abdominal pain and vomiting. Her past medical history includes angioplasty to the left anterior descending artery 10 years earlier, and also to the right coronary artery five years previously. This is her abdominal X-ray.

What does it show?
What is the diagnosis?

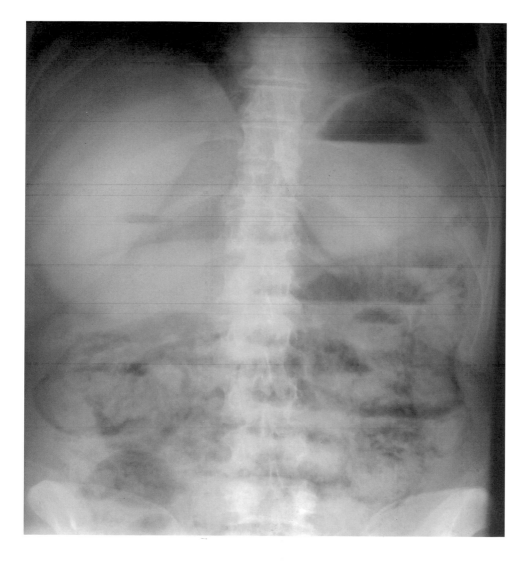

22   This is a barium meal study in a 40-year-old woman with anaemia and weight loss.

What is the diagnosis?

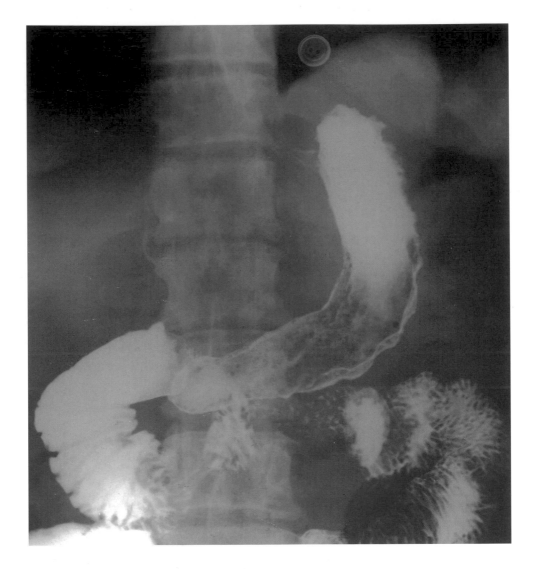

23

A 59-year-old man undergoing investigation for anaemia complains of episodes of vomiting faeculent material, and halitosis. This is a barium study (*see below and overleaf*).

What does it show?

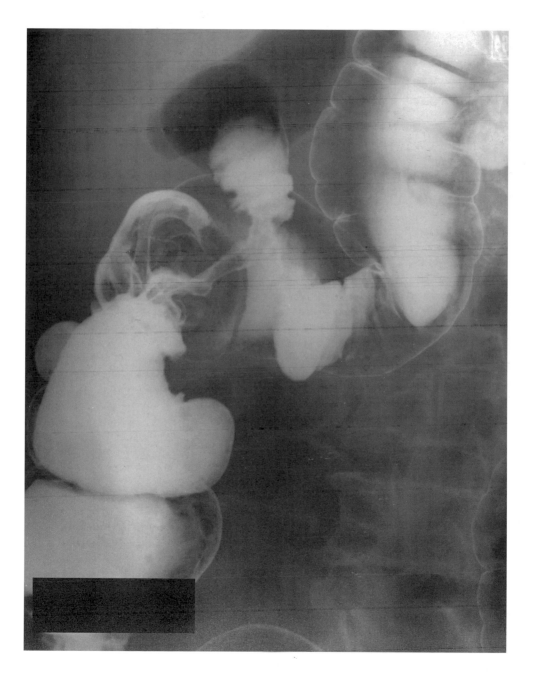

23

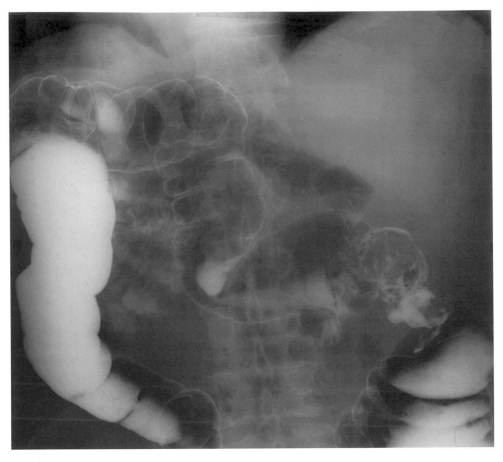

24   A 40-year-old man has undergone biliary surgery for gallstones.
Two weeks later, he complains of right upper quadrant pain and a
fever. This is his X-ray.

What does it show?
What is the diagnosis?

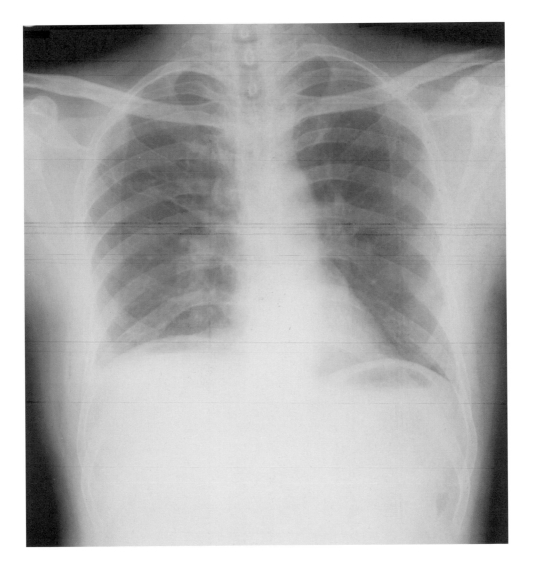

Haematology

1

A 25-year-old man presents with a two-month history of night sweats and weight loss. On examination, he has an erythematous rash in a dermatomal distribution. His Hb is 10.5 g/dL, WCC is 8.2×10^9/L, PLTs are 252×10^9/L.

What does the CXR show?
What is the likely diagnosis?
Name two tests of prognostic value.

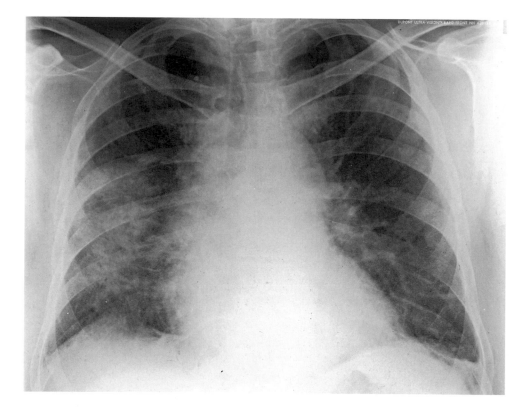

2

This is an X-ray of an 18-year-old boy.

What does the X-ray show?
What is the diagnosis?
How can the diagnosis be confirmed?

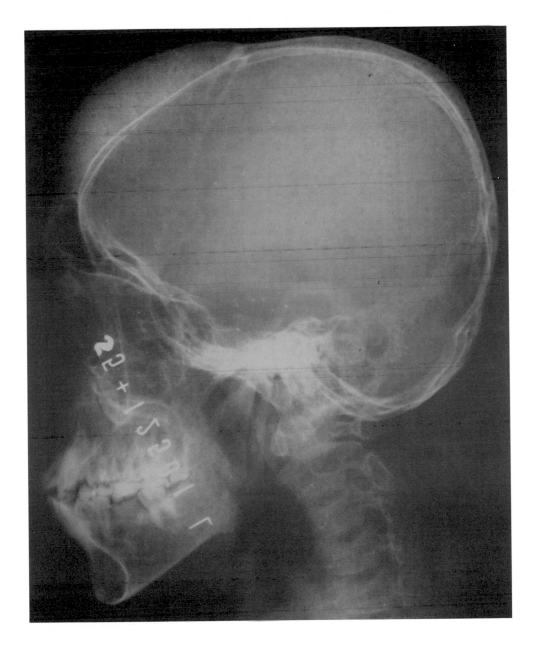

3 These are X-rays of a teenage boy who has regular blood transfusions (*see below and opposite*).

What do the X-rays show?
What is the likely diagnosis?
He was found to have significant glycosuria. Name a possible cause for the above, and describe how it could have been prevented.

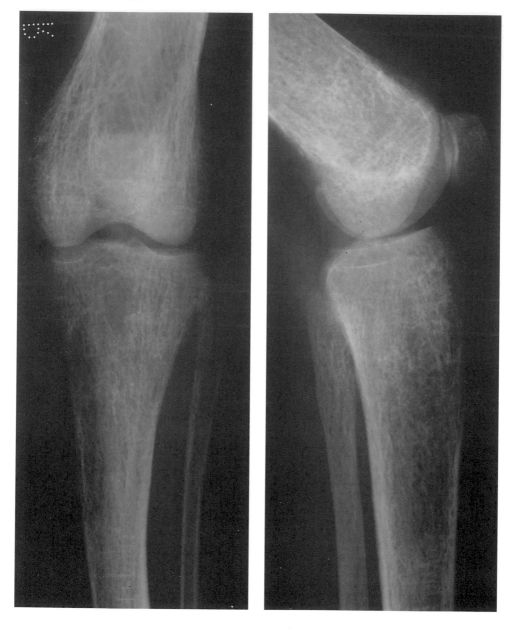

3

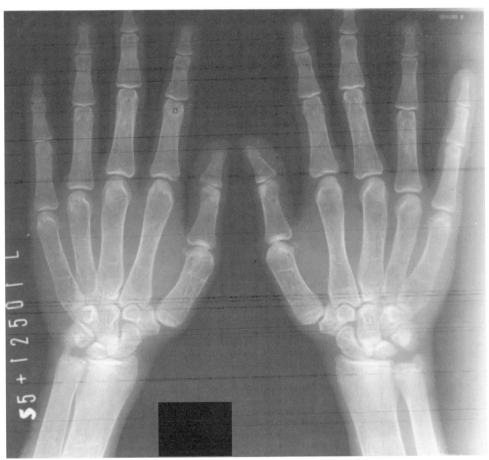

4   A 70-year-old man presents with a chest infection. Routine investigations reveal a plasma viscosity of 2.2, Hb of 8.4 g/dL, WCC of 4.0×10^9/L and platelets of 160×10^9/L. This is his X-ray.

What does it show?
What is the diagnosis?
Name two tests to confirm your suspicions.

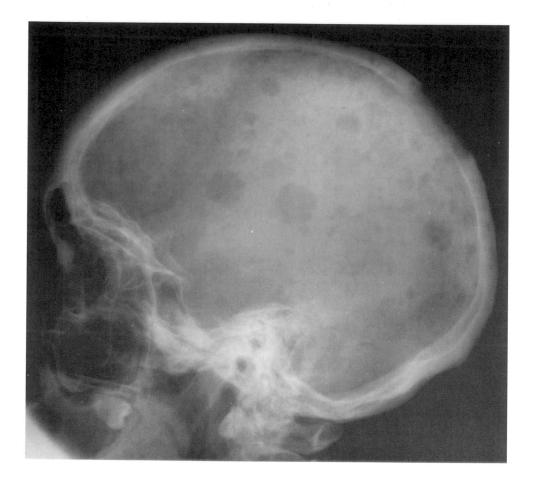

5

A 30-year-old man is admitted to the accident and emergency department unconscious, with evidence of chronic liver disease. Both knees are swollen and deformed, and there are venepuncture scars in both antecubital fossae. Blood tests reveal abnormal LFTs, a normal FBC and an increased APTT but normal PT.

What does this X-ray show?
What is the diagnosis?
Which two complications have occurred as a result of his condition?

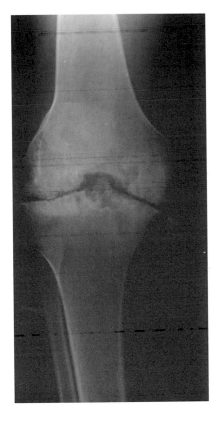
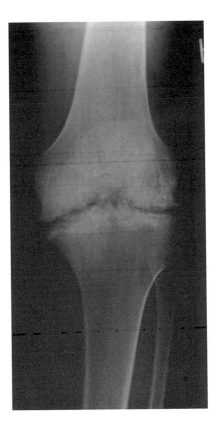

6

This is an MRI scan of a 30-year-old West Indian man (*see below and opposite*).

What does it show?
Give two possible aetiologies for the above.

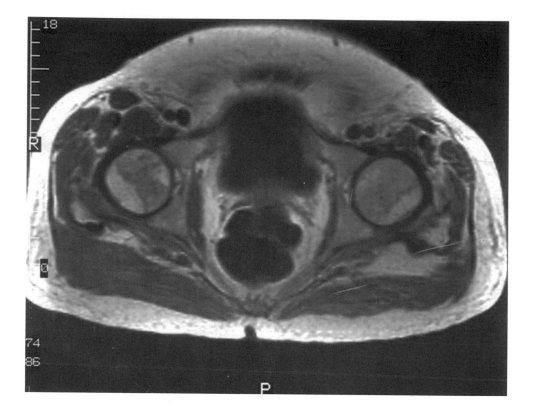

6

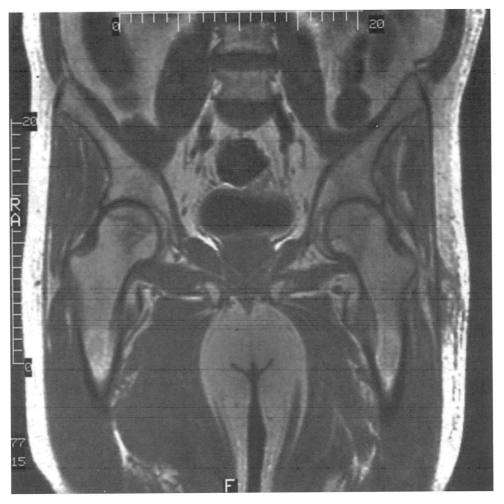

Neurology

1

A 40-year-old woman complains of progressive difficulty in walking. On direct questioning, she admits to difficulty in holding objects, and inspection of her hands reveals several cuts and a large burn over her right hand. This is an MRI scan of the same woman.

What does it show?
What is the diagnosis?

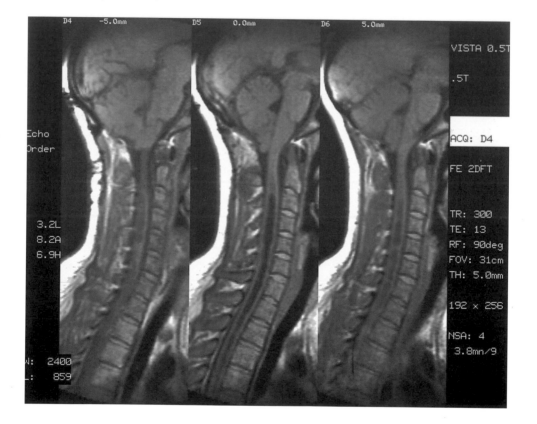

2 A 70-year-old man is found by his granddaughter to be gradually getting more forgetful. Unable to cope alone, he is admitted to hospital. This is a CT scan of his head.

What does it show?

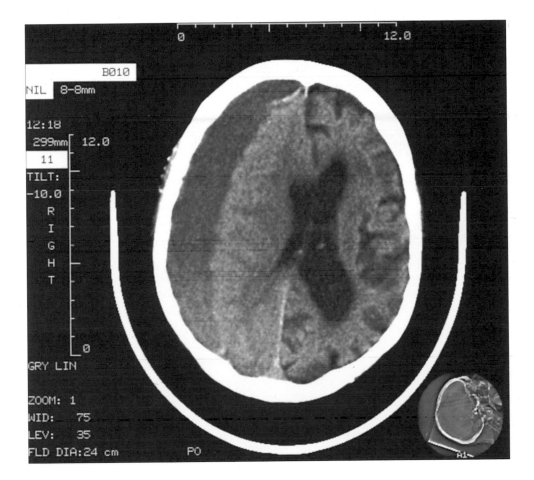

3

A 45-year-old man with a long history of alcohol abuse presented with an acute onset of headaches and mild neck stiffness. Forty-eight hours after admission, he develops fever, marked confusion and agitation. There was no focal neurology of note. A lumbar puncture is carried out, which shows a polymorphonuclear leucocytosis of 5.5×10^3, but no organisms are seen. This is a CT scan of his head (*see below and opposite*).

Describe the findings.
What is the diagnosis?

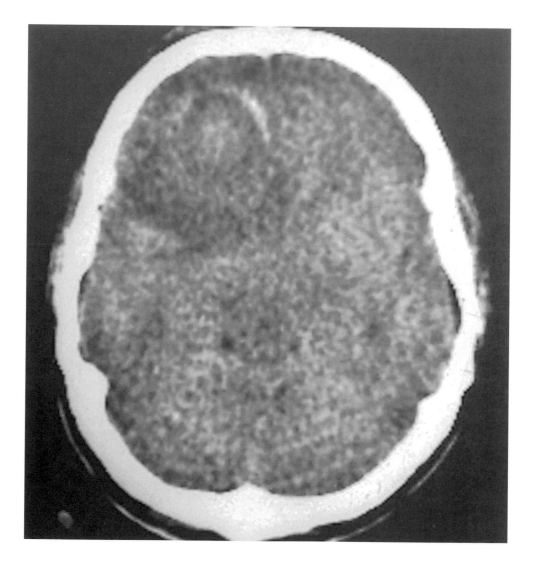

3

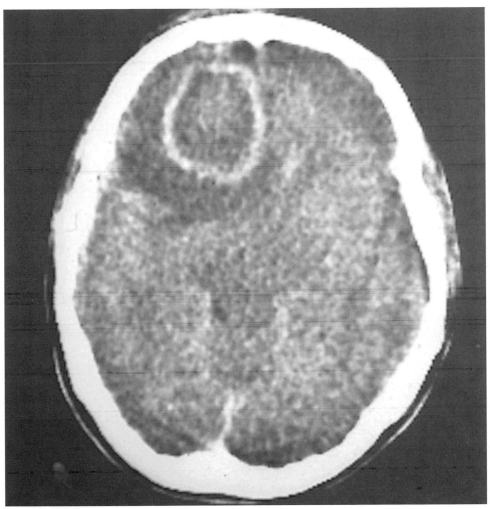

4   A 25-year-old man complains of increasingly frequent fits. The following test is done (*see below and opposite*).

What is the test shown?
Give the diagnosis.
Suggest a possible curative treatment.

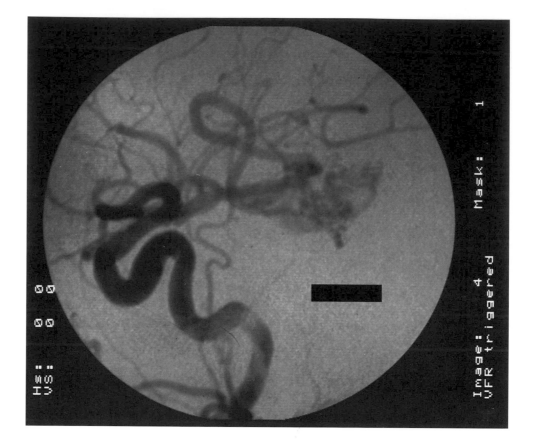

4

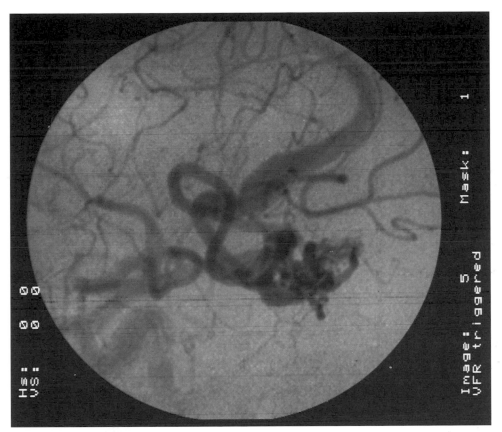

5

A 50-year-old man presents with a three-day history of headaches, nausea and vomiting. His past medical history includes haematuria. After initial tests, he undergoes the following investigations (*see below, opposite and p. 102*).

What do the tests show?
What is the diagnosis?
What is the association between his presentation and the haematuria?

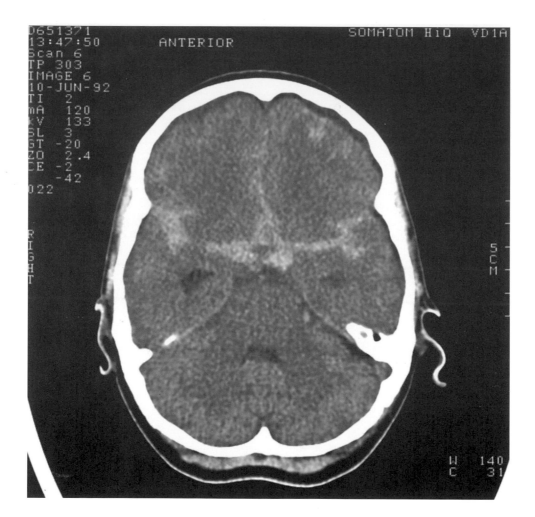

5

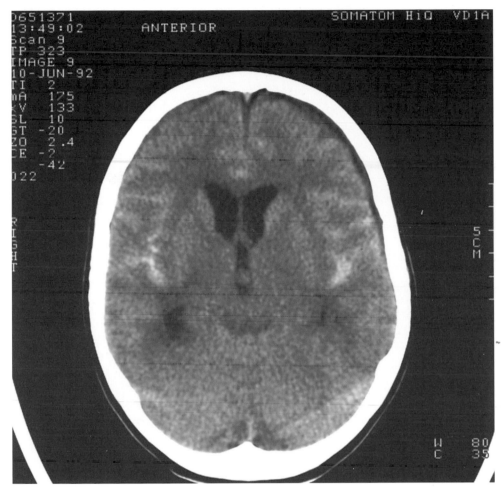

5

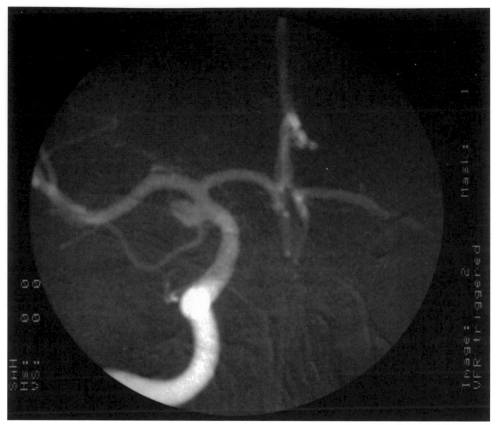

6   This is the skull X-ray of a 24-year-old man with epilepsy.

What does it show?
What is the diagnosis?

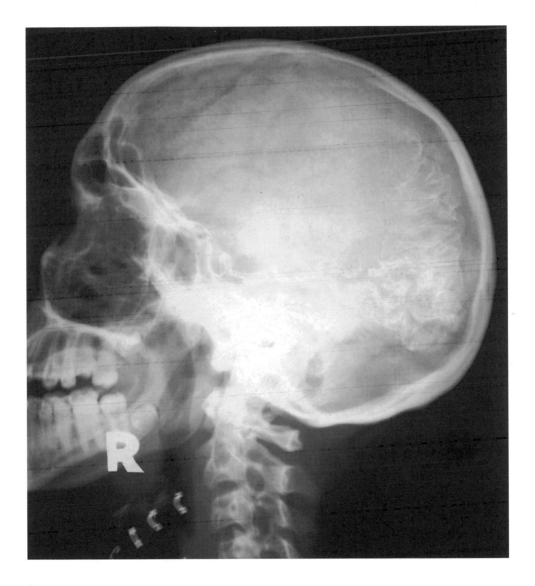

7 These are CT scans of the head of a 48-year-old man with partial seizures (*see below and opposite*).

What do they show?
What is the diagnosis?

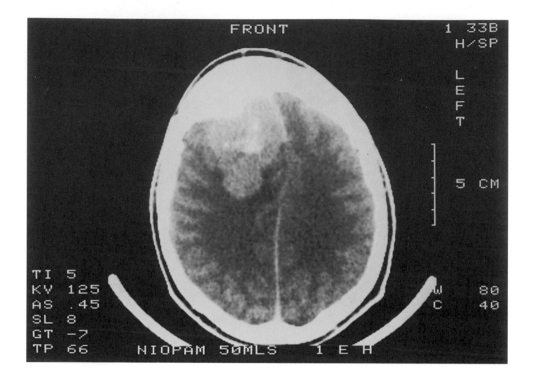

7

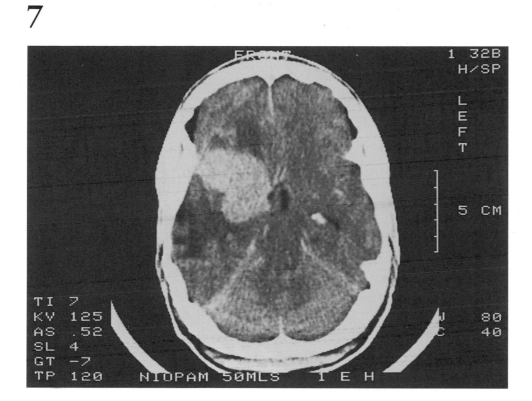

8

A 60-year-old man complains of increasing clumsiness. On examination, he has a number of cuts on both sides of his face, which he says are from shaving. Examination reveals an intention tremor and past-pointing bilaterally. This is an MRI of his head.

What does it show?
What is the diagnosis?

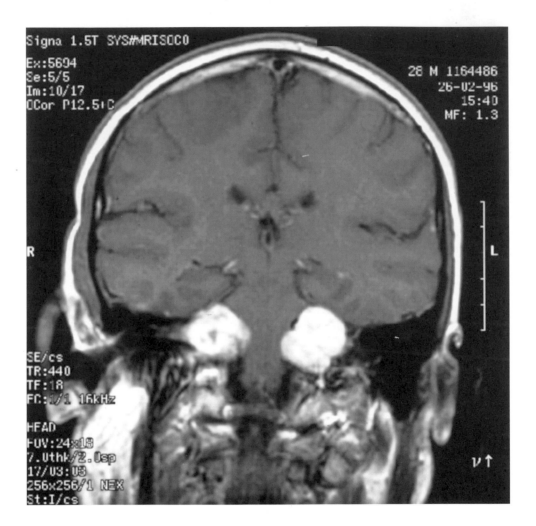

9   This is an MRI scan of a 40-year-old woman with weakness in her legs.

What does it show?
What is the diagnosis?

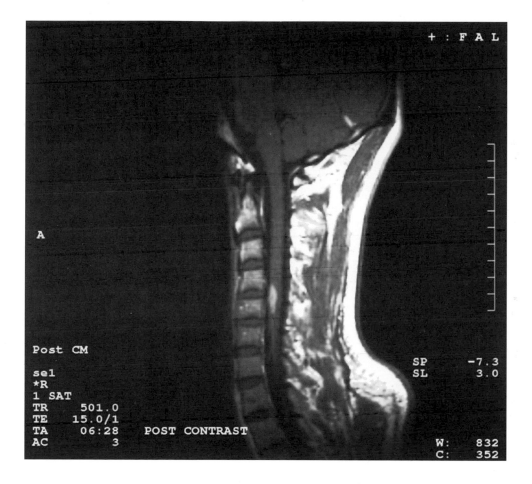

10

A 16-year-old boy with learning difficulties presents to the accident and emergency department with a fit. His mother says that her son has had epilepsy since childhood, but his fits have been increasing in frequency. Neurological examination reveals bilateral brisk reflexes and bilateral extensor plantar responses.

What does the CT show?
What is the diagnosis?
What might you find on the skin?

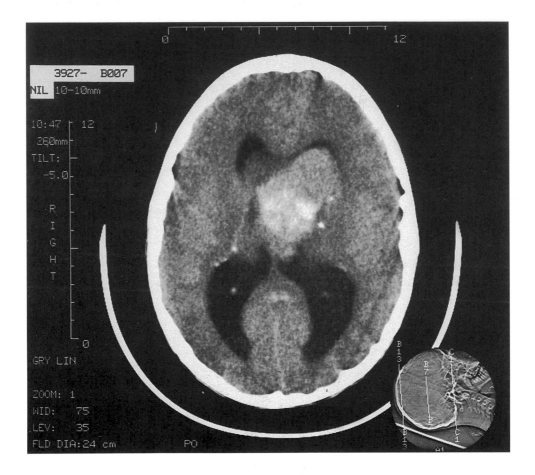

11

A 40-year-old woman develops severe diarrhoea following an episode of *Salmonella* gastroenteritis. Four days later she is admitted, complaining of marked headache. The only abnormality on examination is bilateral papilloedema. Overnight, she spikes a temperature and her conscious level becomes more depressed. An urgent CT scan of her head is organized (*see below, overleaf and p. 111, top*).

What does it show?
Which test is shown at the bottom of p. 111 and what does it show?
What is the diagnosis?

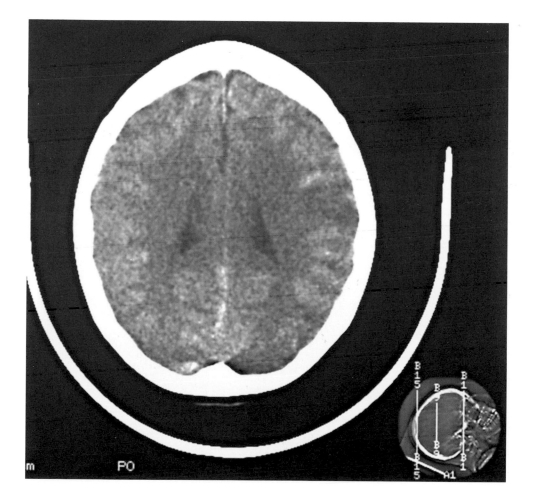

11

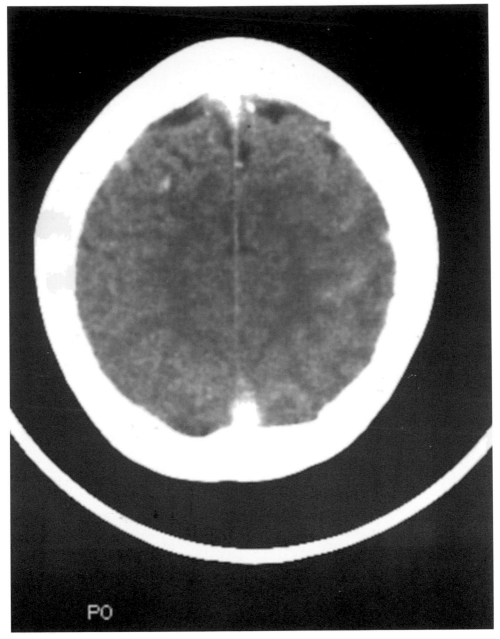

11

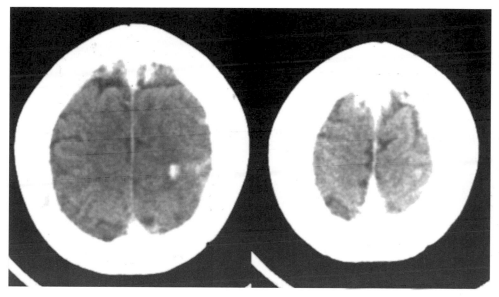

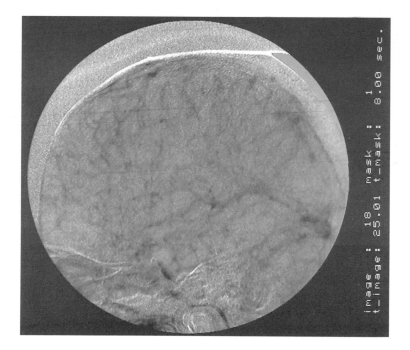

12
This is a CT scan of the head (*see below and opposite*) of a 30-year-old man with headaches. He complains of weight loss and a sore tongue. The examination reveals generalized lymphadenopathy, *Candida* on the tongue and needle marks on his arm.

What do the scans show?
What is the diagnosis?
How would you confirm the diagnosis?

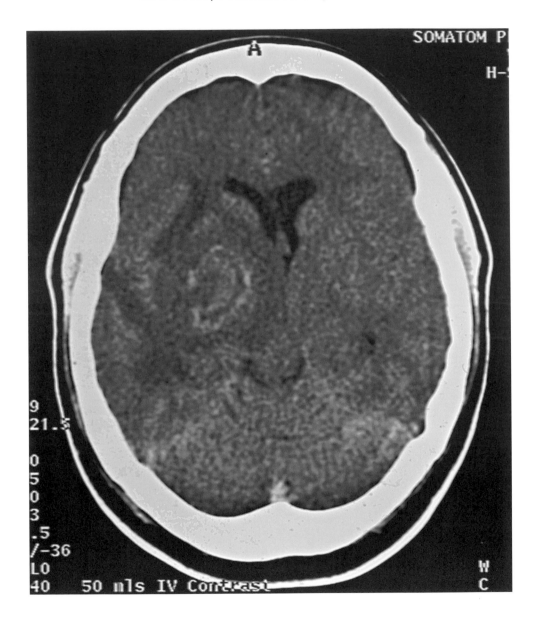

12

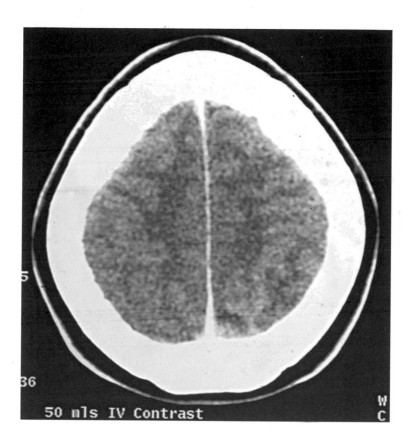

50 mls IV Contrast

13

A 40-year-old man complains of unilateral swelling of his left eye. He had been intoxicated and had fallen the night before. The following test is done.

What does it show?
Which complications can occur?
How might it be treated?

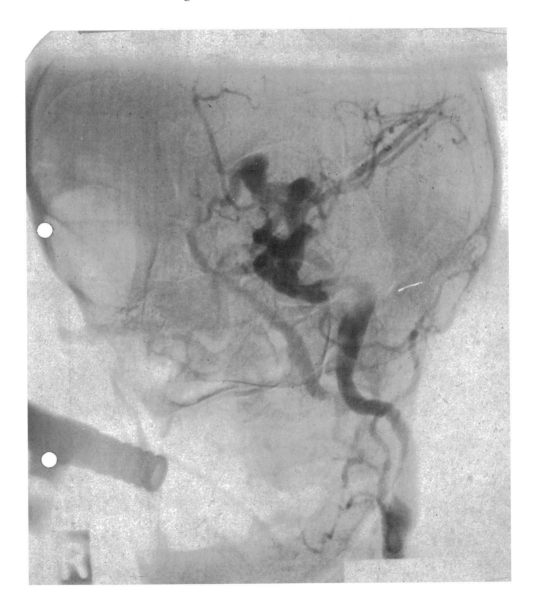

14 A 70-year-old woman presents with a four-day history of feeling generally unwell and drowsy. She is found to be pyrexial with a temperature of 41 °C. Blood, urine and sputum cultures are all negative. The patient becomes more confused, and develops a unilateral motor deficit in her lower limbs. This is a CT scan of her head.

What does it show?
Which other non-invasive test may be helpful?
What is the likely diagnosis?

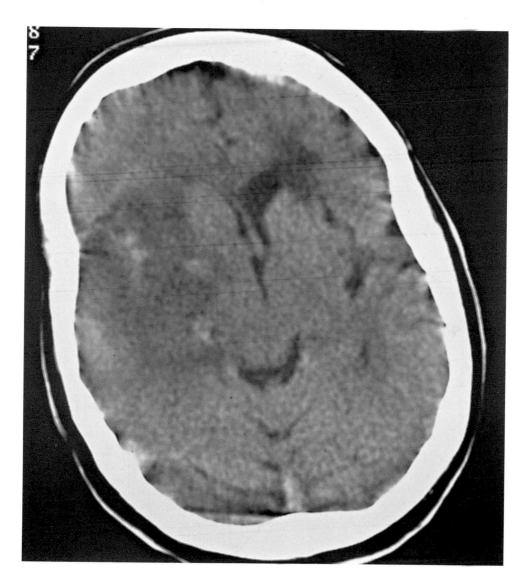

Renal

1   What does the radiograph show?
Which complications can occur?

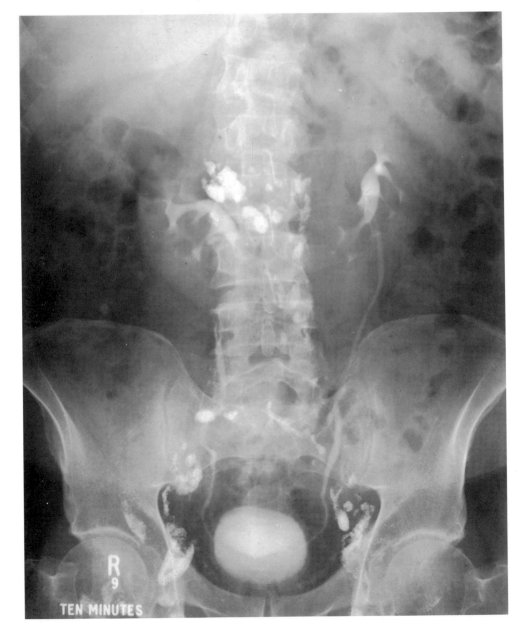

R
9
TEN MINUTES

2   A 40-year-old man complains of loin pain and haematuria. This is a scan of the abdomen (*see below and overleaf*).

What do the scans show?
What is the diagnosis?
Which other forms of renal disease are associated with this?

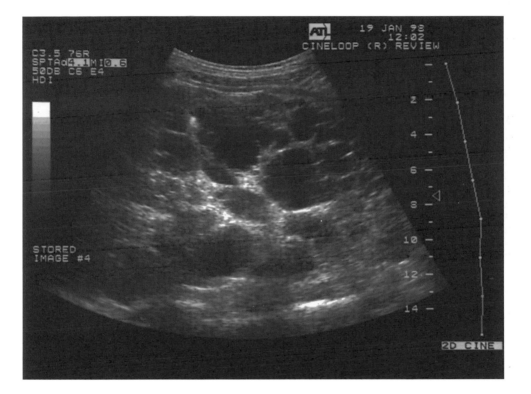

2

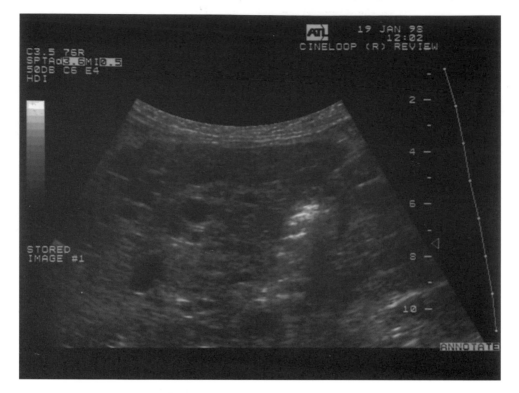

3 A 50-year-old woman presented with lethargy, weight loss and shortness of breath. Investigations revealed anaemia and moderate renal impairment. This is her IVU.

What does it show?
What is the underlying cause of the renal impairment?

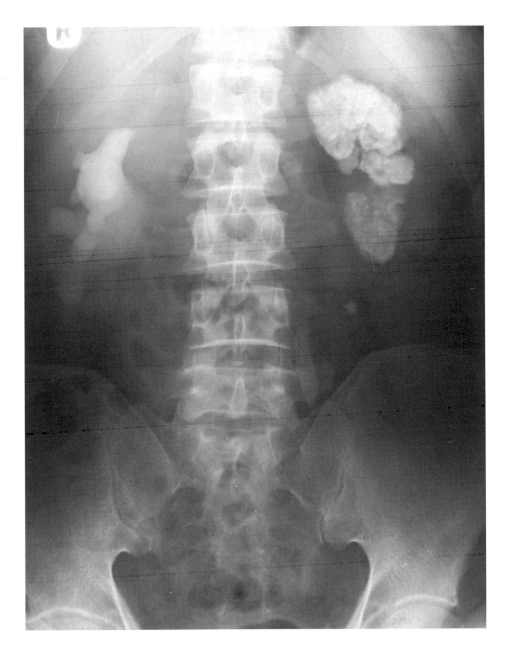

4

A 31-year-old man presented with a two-month history of weight loss and three days of abdominal pain. He was investigated by gastroscopy and a US scan of the abdomen, both of which were normal. He subsequently developed a stroke. Investigations revealed a normocytic normochromic anaemia, a high acute-phase response, abnormal LFTs and microscopic haematuria. The following investigation was done initially (*see below*) and then repeated 3 months later (*see opposite*).

Which investigations are shown?
Describe the radiological findings and what is the diagnosis?
Give two possible causes of the stroke.
What are the other neurological manifestations of this condition?

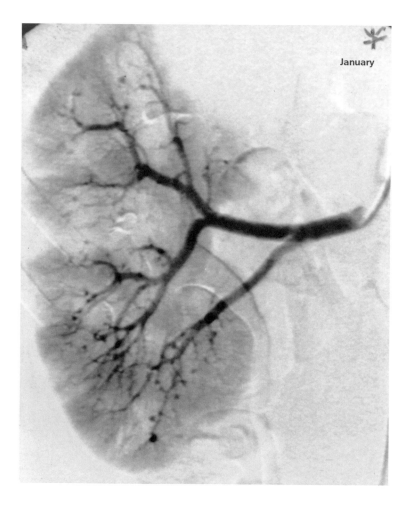

January

4

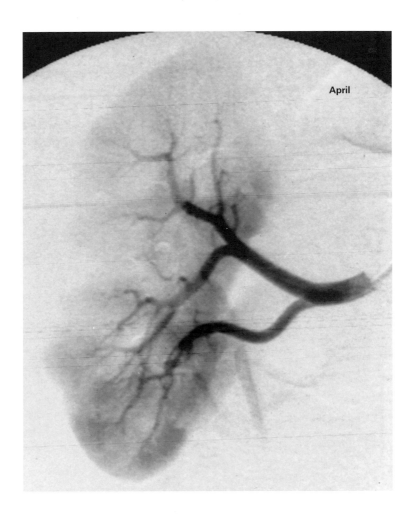

April

5   A 60-year-old woman with sarcoidosis presented with fever and dysuria. Over the preceding five years, she had had recurrent episodes of loin pain and urinary tract infections. This is an AXR.

What does it show?
What is the likely cause of the abnormality shown?

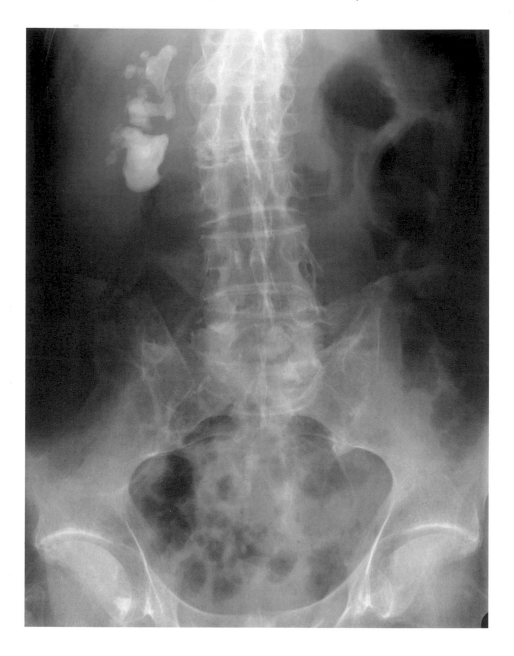

6 A 70-year-old man complains of a one-year history of tiredness, polyuria and polydipsia. On examination, he is plethoric and cachectic, with a palpable abdominal mass. His serum calcium is elevated, at 2.95 mmol/L, and he has a urea level of 14 mmol/L and a creatinine level of 150 μmol/L. This is an angiogram of the patient.

What does it show?
What is the diagnosis?
What is the cause of the hypercalcaemia?
What is the patient's Hb level likely to be?
Which other test might you wish to do?

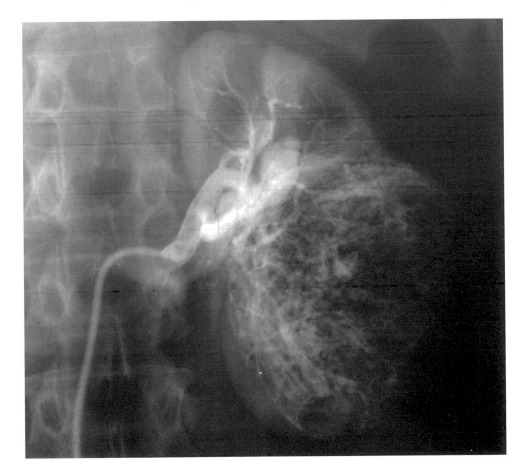

7   A 70-year-old man presents with fever and loin pain. Investigations reveal anaemia, an elevated ESR and moderate renal impairment. The following investigation is done (*see below*).

What does it show?
What is the cause of the renal impairment?

A year later, he complains of hip and back pain. He has the test shown (*see opposite*).

What does it show?
What is the cause of the back pain?

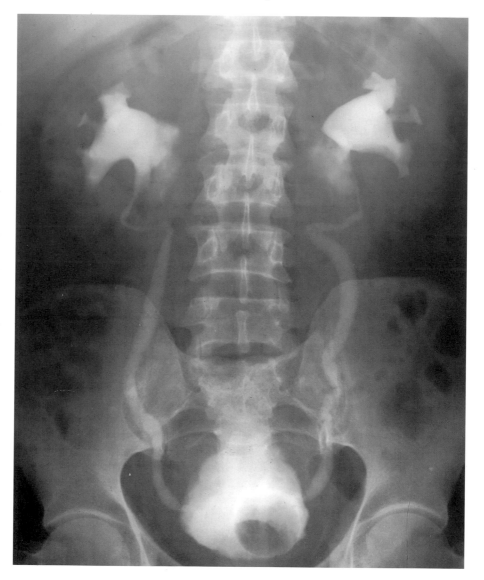

7

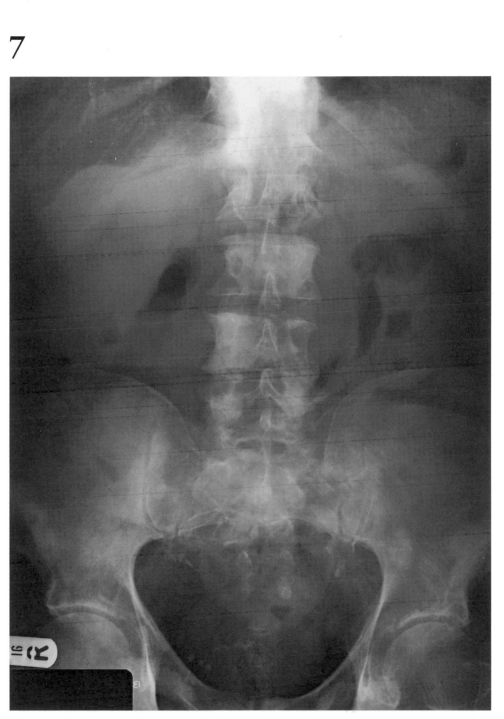

8

This is an X-ray of a woman with loin pain.

Give the likely diagnosis and a possible alternative diagnosis.

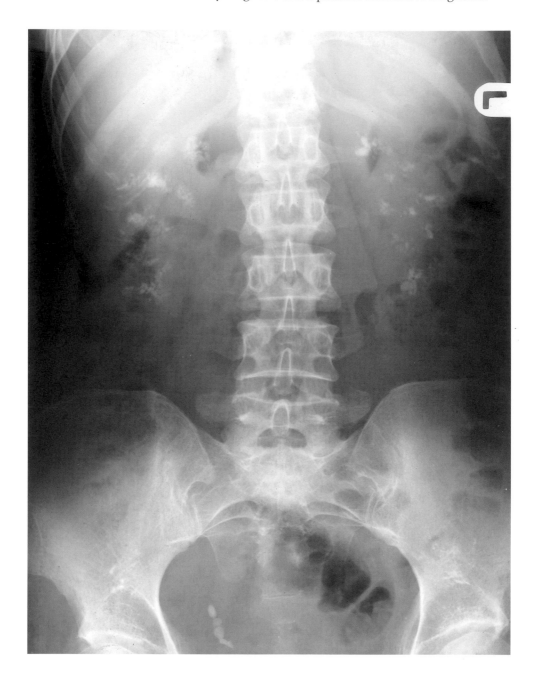

9   A 36-year-old bank manager complains of headaches. He has a number of tests, one of which is shown (*see below and overleaf*).

Which investigation is shown?
What does it show?
What is the diagnosis?

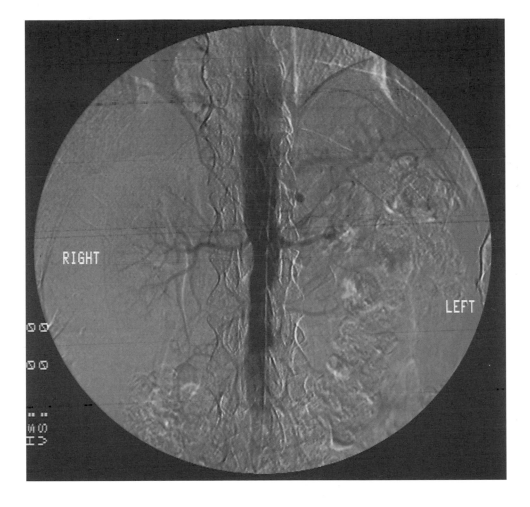

9

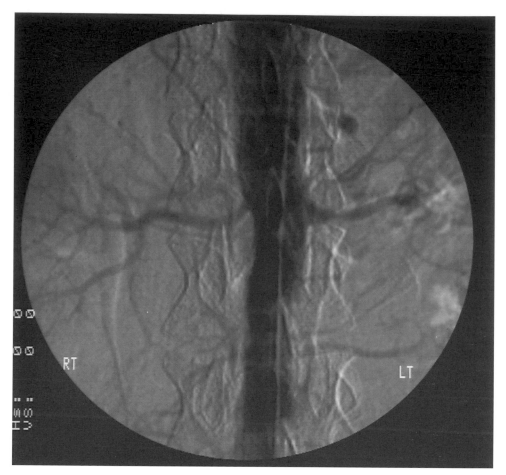

10

A 16-year-old boy complains of headaches. He is found to have a persistently elevated diastolic blood pressure of 100 mmHg. The past medical history includes recurrent episodes of abdominal pain and fever.

Which investigation is shown?
What is the cause of his loin pain?
What is the cause of his hypertension?
How is this condition graded?

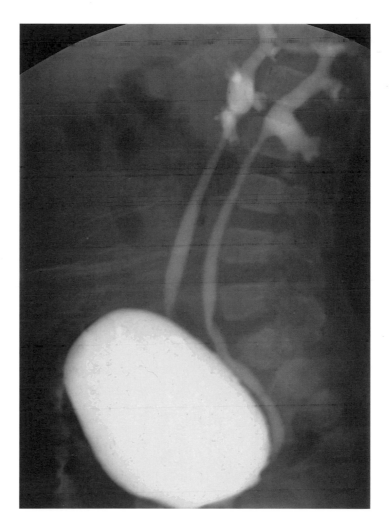

11   This is an IVU of a 46-year-old patient with hypertension and renal impairment.

What is the diagnosis?

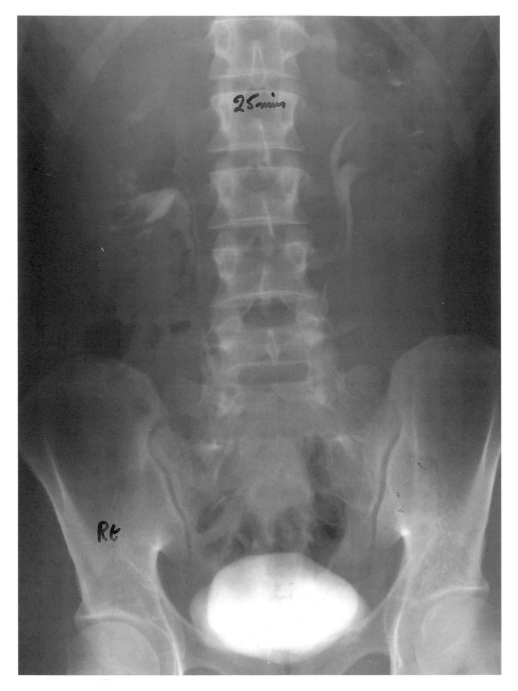

12   This man has difficulty dialysing.

What is the reason?

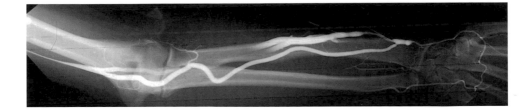

13   These are CT scans of a patient with weight loss (*see below and opposite*).

What do they show?

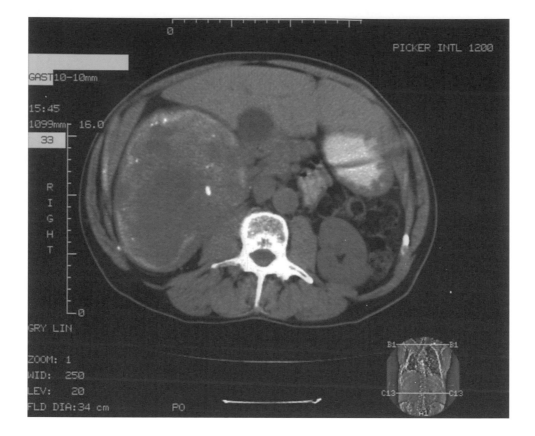

13

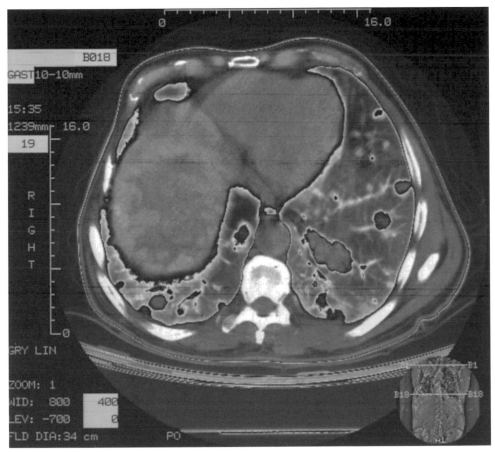

Respiratory Medicine

1   This CXR was taken during a routine health screening examination.

What is the diagnosis?

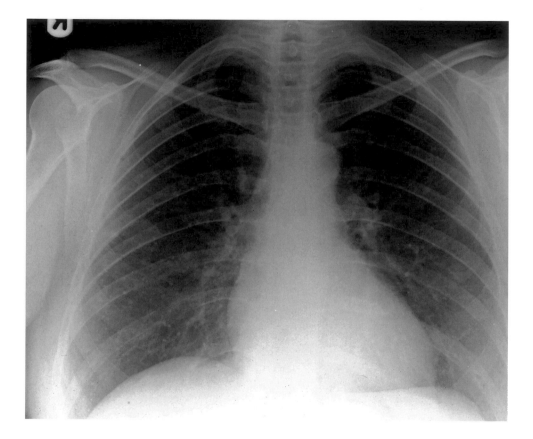

2

This is a radiograph of a 35-year-old patient who has had asthma since childhood. On this occasion, the presenting complaint is fever, shortness of breath and haemoptysis.

What does the X-ray show?
What is the likely cause of the haemoptysis?
What is the likely aetiology of these radiological changes?
Give two tests that might support this diagnosis.

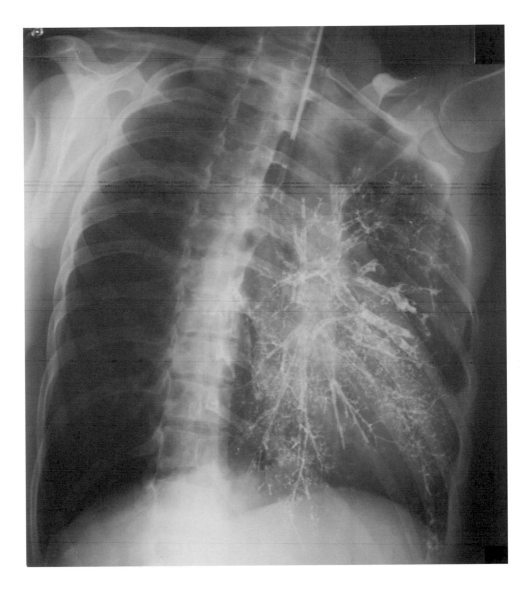

3

This teenager was admitted with intestinal obstruction. He is markedly short of breath, with a fruity cough. His past medical history includes numerous admissions with chest infections. This is a CXR (*see below and opposite*).

What does it show?
What is the likely diagnosis?
How would you confirm the diagnosis?

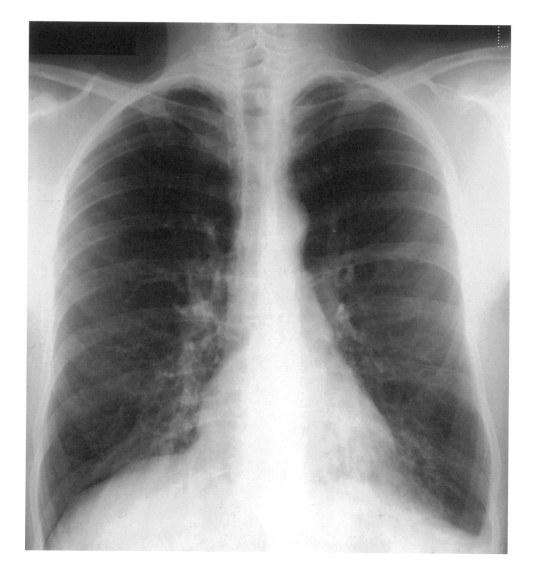

3

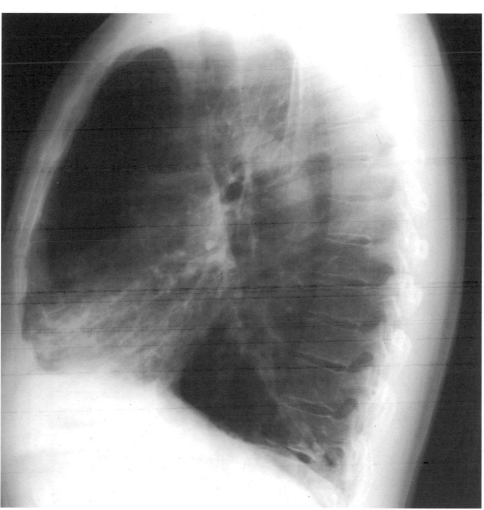

4   This is a CXR of a man presenting with shortness of breath. His spirometry shows a mild obstructive defect.

What does the CXR show?
What is the diagnosis?
What evidence might support the diagnosis?

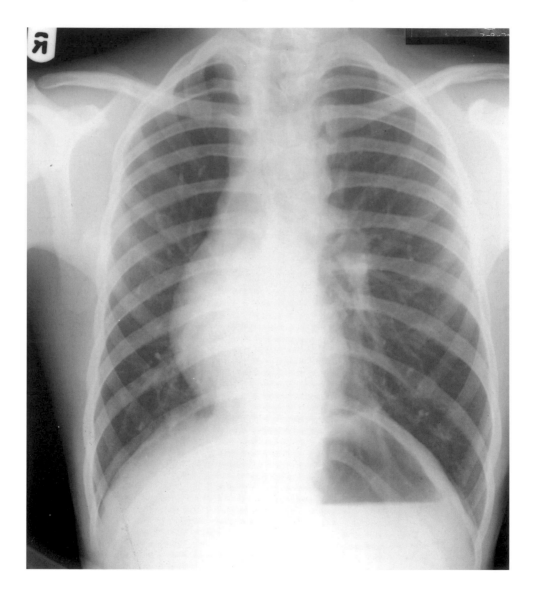

5 An 80-year-old woman complains of pain in her right shoulder and forearm.

What does her CXR show?
What is the diagnosis?
Name three other clinical features that may occur in this condition.

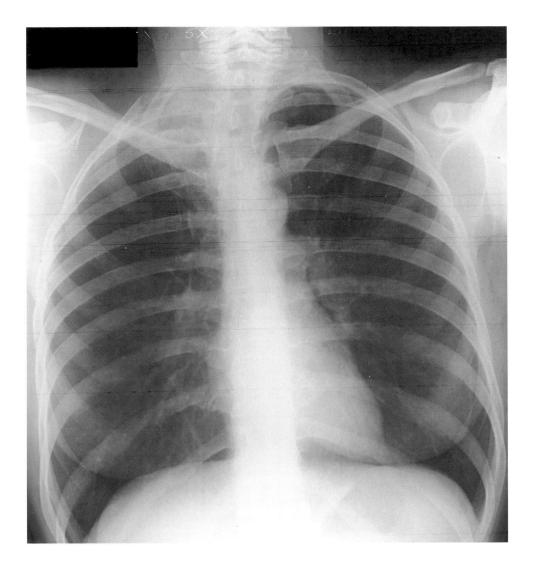

6   A 40-year-old man presents with a one-year history of dry cough. Recently, he has noticed increasing amounts of haemoptysis, which have culminated in an admission to hospital.

What does his CXR show?
What is the diagnosis?
How can the diagnosis be confirmed?
What are the treatment options?

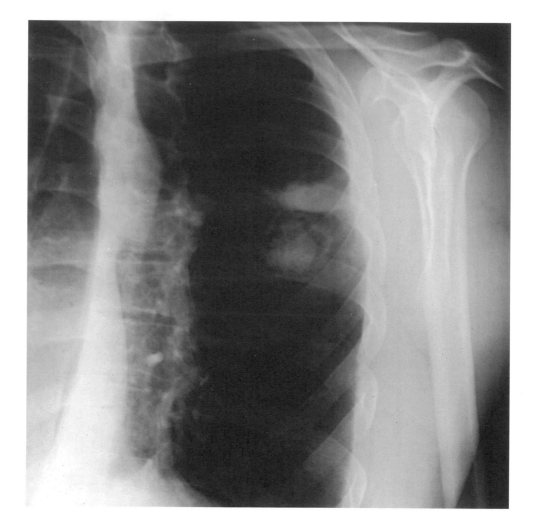

7   A 28-year-old man complains of painful eyes, hands and face. On examination, he has painful swelling on his hands and over the right side of his face.

What does his CXR show?
What is the diagnosis?
Which tests could you do to confirm the diagnosis?
Name the syndrome.

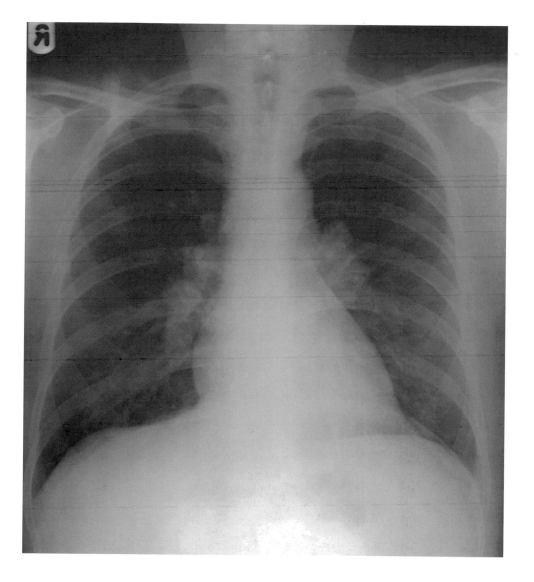

8   This CXR was carried out in an asymptomatic 40-year-old non-smoker during a routine medical examination at work.

What does the CXR show?
What is the probable diagnosis?

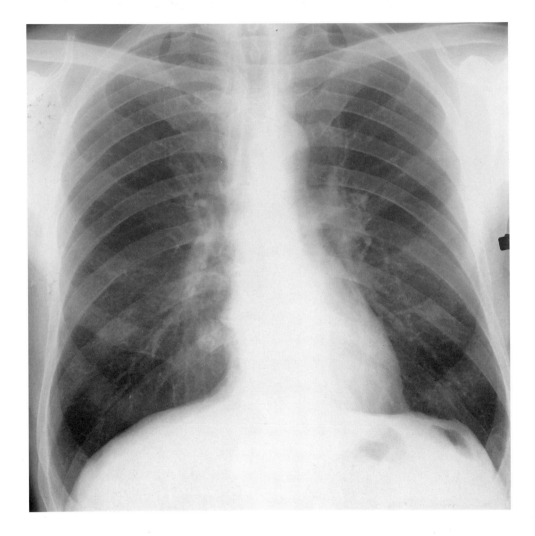

9   A 25-year-old heroin addict presents to the admissions unit feeling generally unwell, and complaining of chest pain and feeling feverish. He has recently completed a course of antibiotics for a suspected chest infection. On examination, he has pyrexia of 38°C, prominent venous pulsation in the neck, a loud pansystolic murmur at the left sternal edge and an enlarged, pulsatile liver.

What does the CXR show?
What is the diagnosis?
Which tests would you perform to confirm your diagnosis?

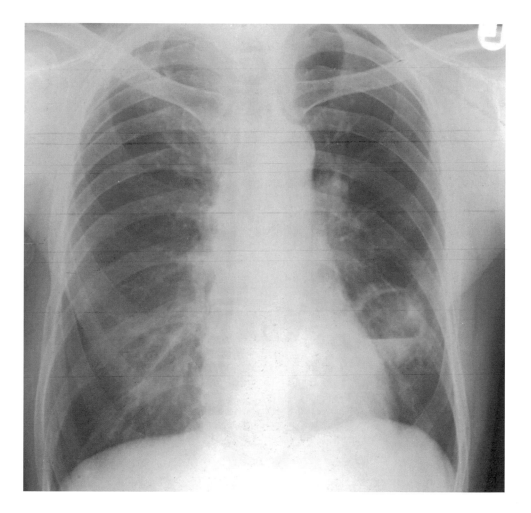

10

A 50-year-old self-employed plumber with asthma has taken early retirement due to progressive breathlessness. Three years later, he complains of increasing breathlessness and chest pain. This is his CXR.

What is the diagnosis?
What is the likely aetiology of his condition?

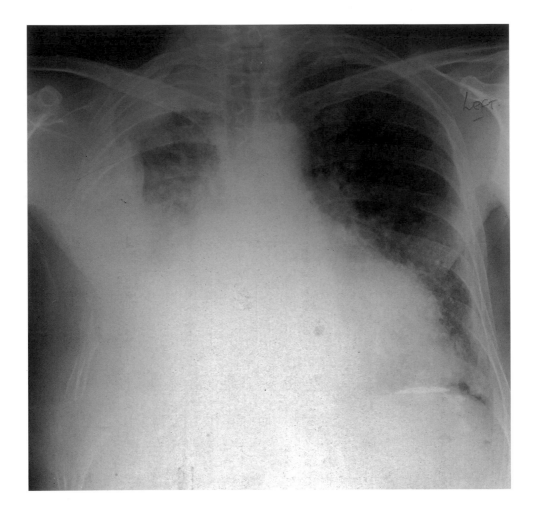

11

A 58-year-old man complains of breathlessness. His CXR shows mild reticular shadowing, but little else. His lung function tests show a mild restrictive defect, with a slight reduction in transfer factor. Several years later, he becomes housebound. Repeat lung function tests show a reduction in lung volume and a further reduction in transfer factor.

What does the CXR show now?
What is the diagnosis?

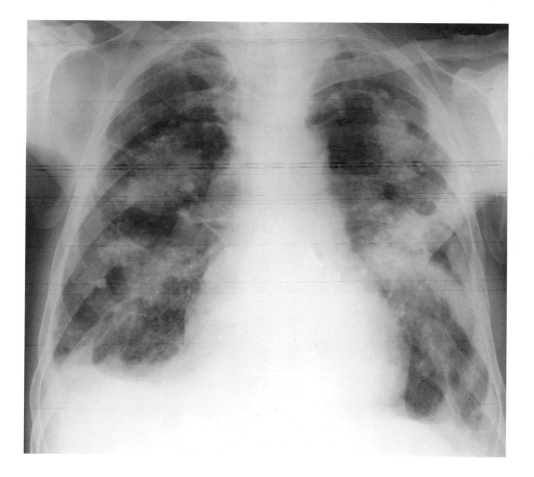

12

A 42-year-old man complains of a cough and recurrent haemoptysis. His CXR is unremarkable, and his symptoms remit. He later develops swelling of his ankles and hands. His urea is 24 mmol/L and his creatinine is 240 μmol/L. Urine microscopy shows red cell casts. A CXR is performed, as he again complains of haemoptysis as well as intermittent epistaxis.

What does the CXR show?
What is the diagnosis?
Which tests would you do to confirm the diagnosis?

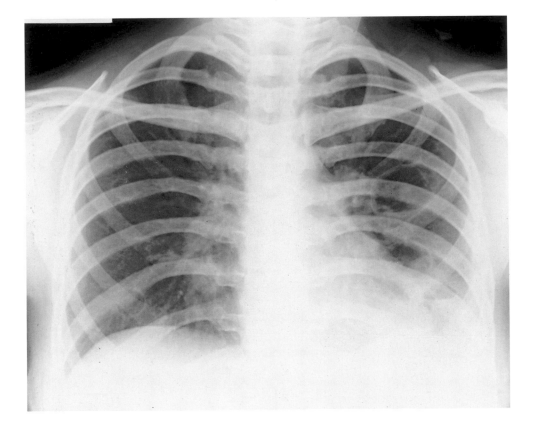

13   This is a CXR of a 54-year-old man with shortness of breath.

What does it show?

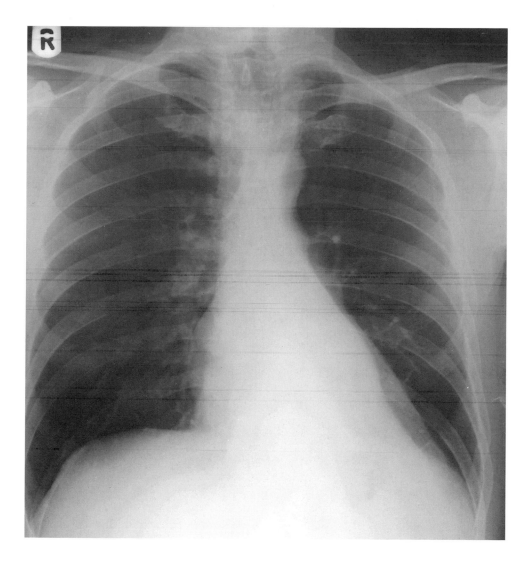

14   A 60-year-old woman presents to her general practitioner with a one-month history of headaches and progressive swelling of her hands. She also complains of an eight-month history of weight loss. Two tests are shown (*see below and opposite*).

What does each show?
What is the diagnosis?

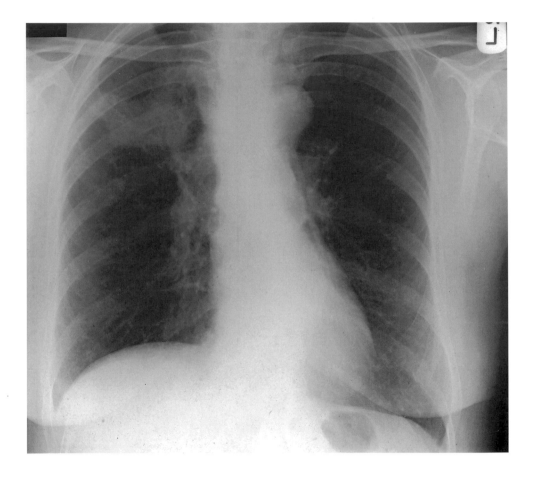

14

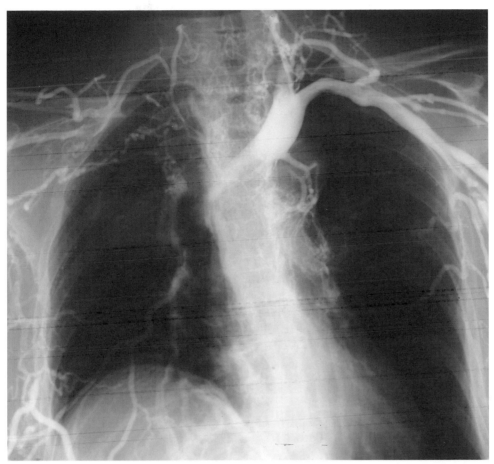

15

A 20-year-old man complains of lethargy, shortness of breath and double vision. This is his CXR.

What does it show?
What is the diagnosis?
Which test would you do to confirm the diagnosis?

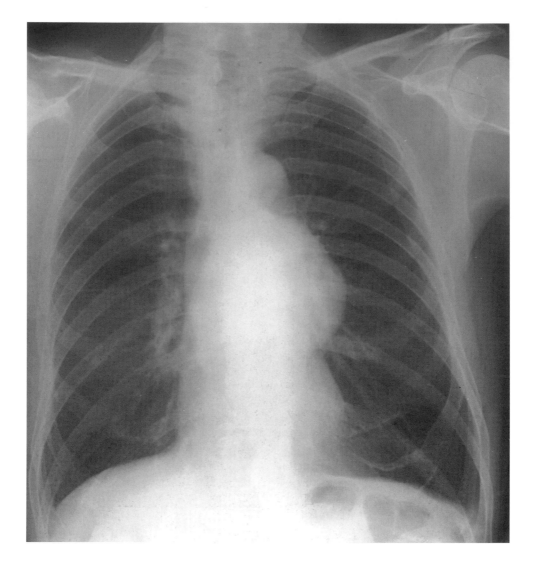

16   This is a CXR of a man who has been involved in a road traffic accident.

Which abnormalities are shown?
What would you expect to find on auscultation of the heart?

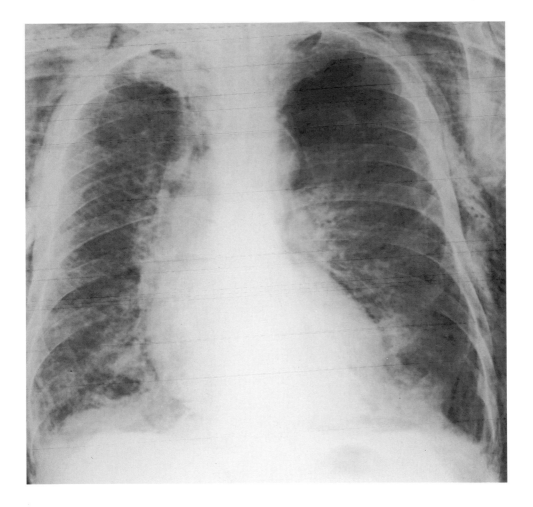

17   A 24-year-old woman undergoing investigation for renal impairment and arthritis has become acutely dyspnoeic. She subsequently has a cardiorespiratory arrest and is successfully resuscitated. She is supported on intensive care overnight, and the below test is done the following day.

What does it show?
Which blood tests would you consider doing in this woman?
What is the unifying diagnosis?

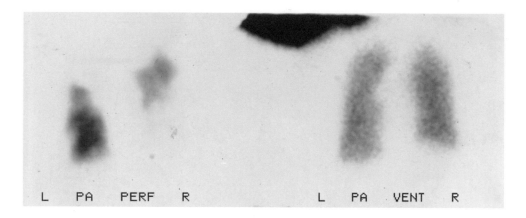

Skeletal

1 A 60-year-old woman complains of pain and difficulty with holding objects in her hands. This is an X-ray of her hands.

What does it show?
What is the diagnosis?

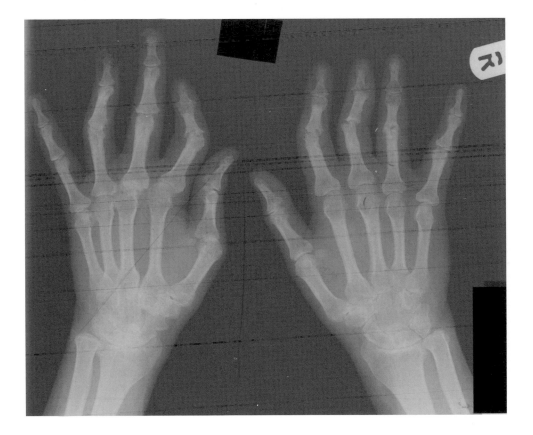

2   This is the X-ray of a 65-year-old man who presented with a sudden onset of pain and swelling of the knee joint (*see below and opposite*).

What does it show?
What is the diagnosis?
How can the diagnosis be confirmed, and which other tests may be useful here?

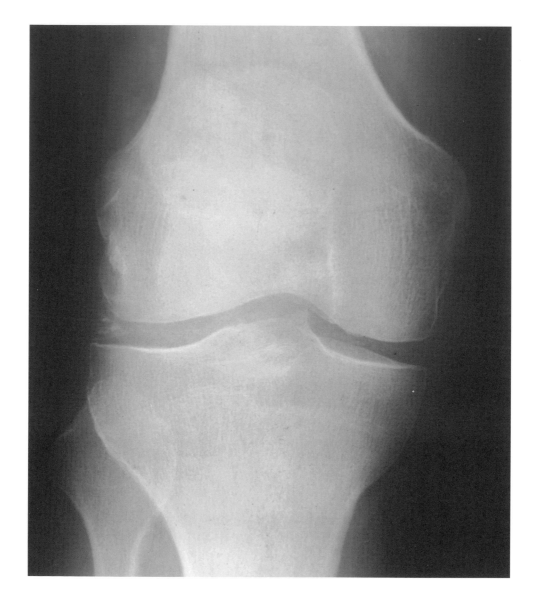

2

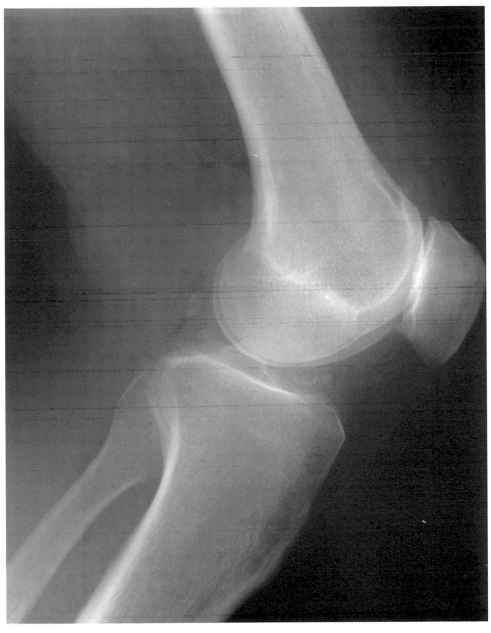

3 A 64-year-old woman complains of painful hands. This is an X-ray of her hands.

What does the X-ray show?
Which other symptoms might you expect?
What might you find on inspection?
What is the diagnosis?

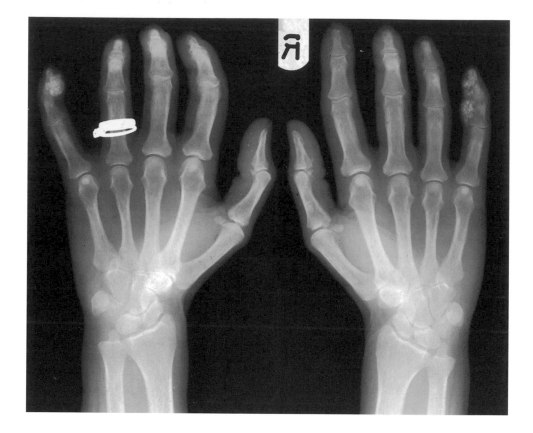

4   A 40-year-old Asian woman with a long history of diarrhoea and dermatitis herpetiformis complains of back, hip and arm pain. She also complains of difficulty in walking up the stairs.

What do the X-rays show (*see below and overleaf*)?
What is the diagnosis?
Which tests would you do to confirm this?
What is the cause of the difficulty in walking up the stairs?

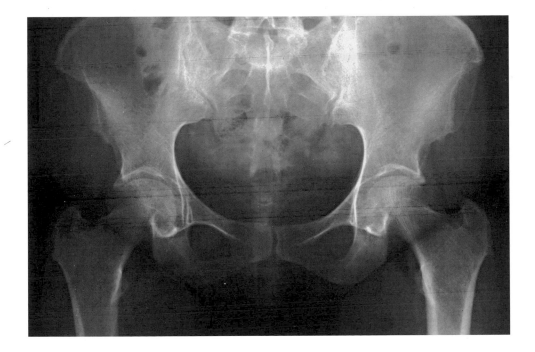

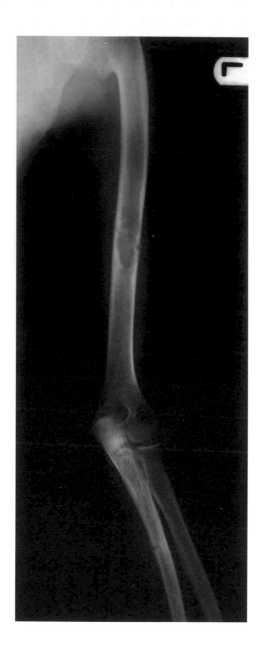

5

These are a CXR and hand X-ray of a patient with a 25-year history of diabetes mellitus, who has ceased regular attendance at the diabetic clinic (*see below and overleaf*).

What do the X-rays show?
What is the diagnosis?
Which biochemical abnormality has led to these radiological changes?

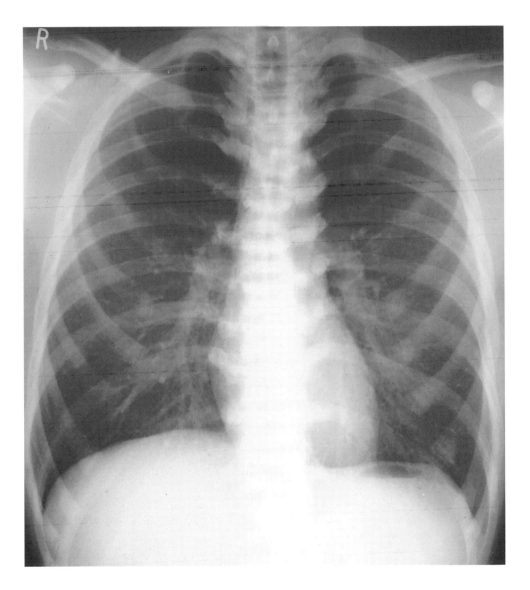

5

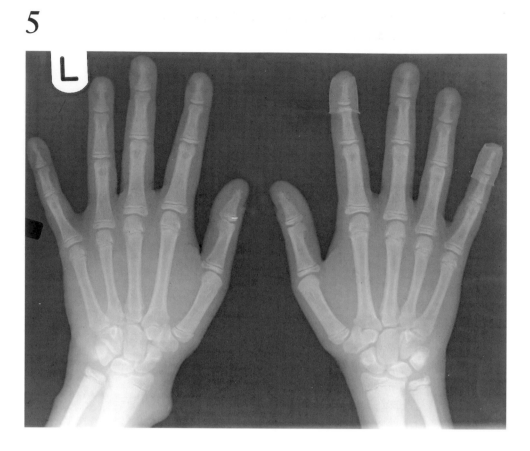

6   This is a skull X-ray of a 75-year-old man who complains of headaches and poor hearing.

What does the X-ray show?
What is the diagnosis?
What are the two likely causes of his deafness?

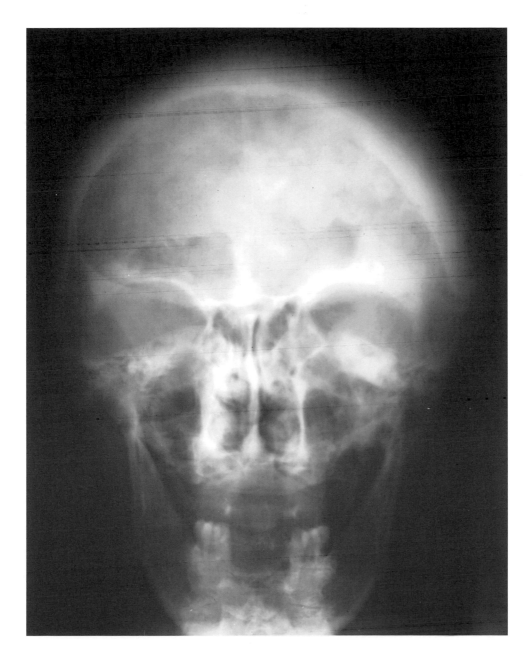

7 A 40-year-old man complains of progressive shortness of breath on exertion. This is an X-ray of his spine (*see below and opposite*).

What does it show?
What is the diagnosis?
What are the possible causes of his breathlessness?
What might his ECG show?

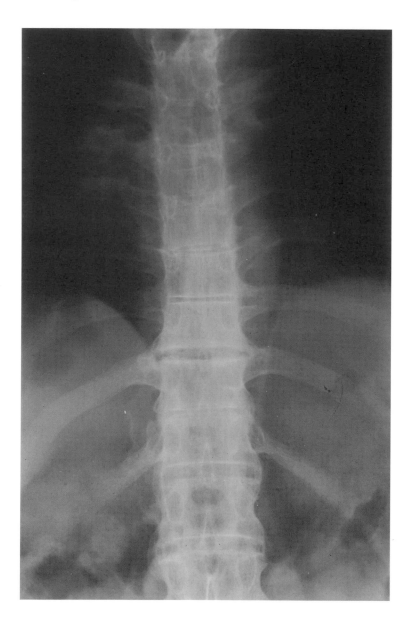

7

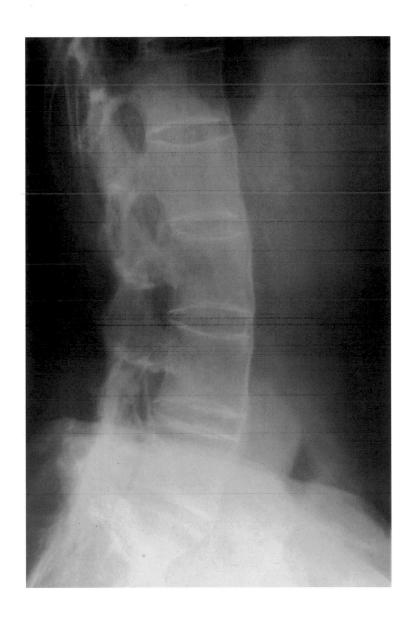

8   A 60-year-old man with poor vision is found to have a painless
     ulcer on his foot. These are his X-rays (*see below and opposite*).

     What do they show?
     Which tests are mandatory?
     If these tests turn out to be negative, what are the other possible
     diagnoses?

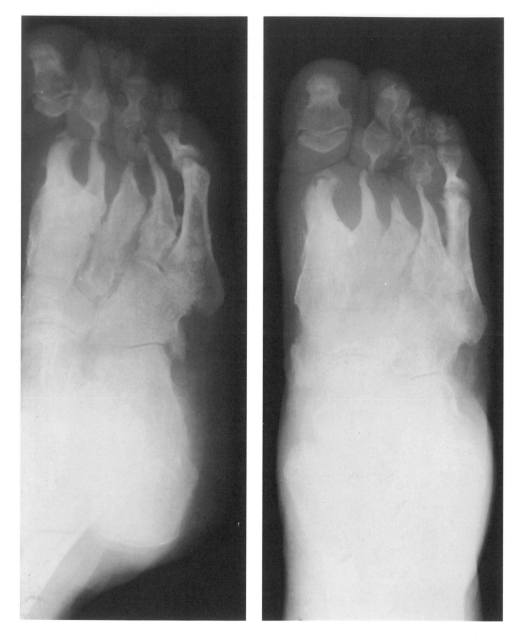

8

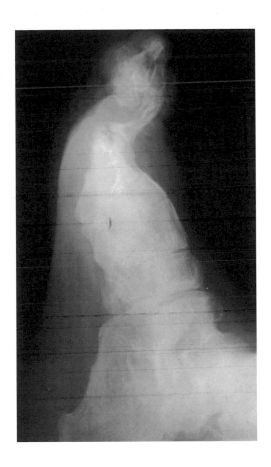

9

A 65-year-old woman complains of painful hands and feet. This is an X-ray of her hands.

What does it show?
What is the diagnosis?

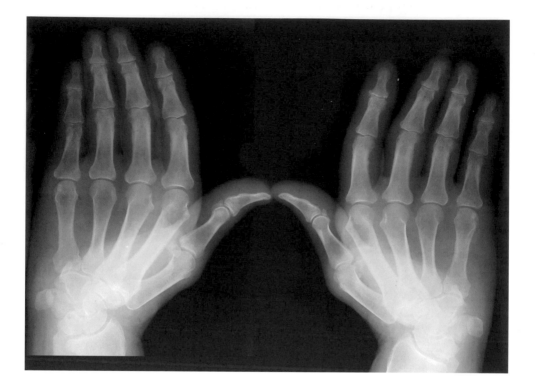

10   This patient complains of a sudden onset of pain and swelling of her calf.

What would a Doppler scan of her calf show?
Which test is shown, and what does it show?
What condition is she suffering from?

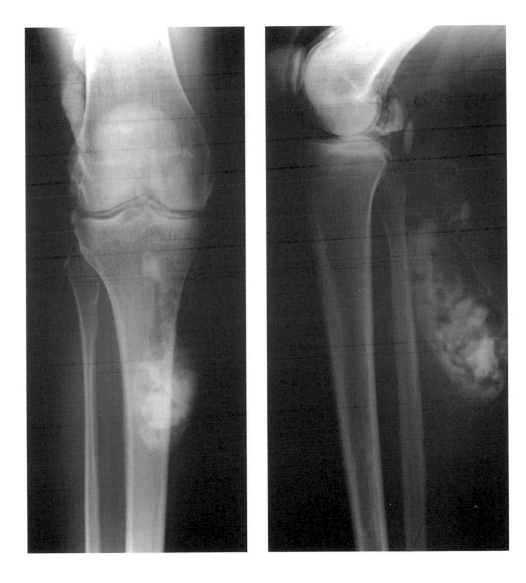

11

A 24-year-old man with severe learning difficulties and behavioural disturbance complains of pain and swelling in his hands. Over the years, he has had similar repeated attacks, which were treated with analgesics. On examination, there is evidence of self-mutilation and a painful, warm, swollen red hand. This is his X-ray.

What does it show?
What is the cause of the pain?
What condition is this man is suffering from?

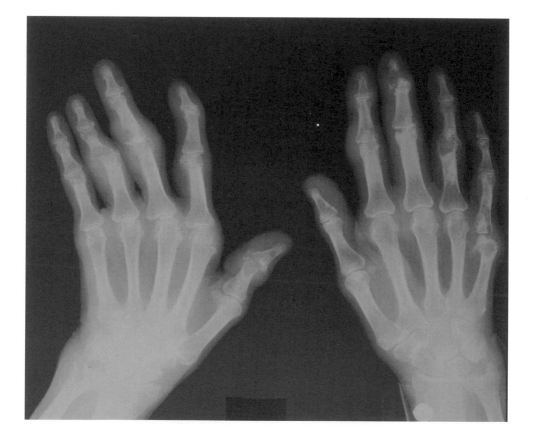

12   A 55-year-old man is admitted with a left lower lobe pneumonia. He has had pneumonia three months earlier in the same territory. He also describes constant backache, which he had attributed to his manual job, for eight months. This is a radionucleotide study.

What does it show?
What is the likely diagnosis?

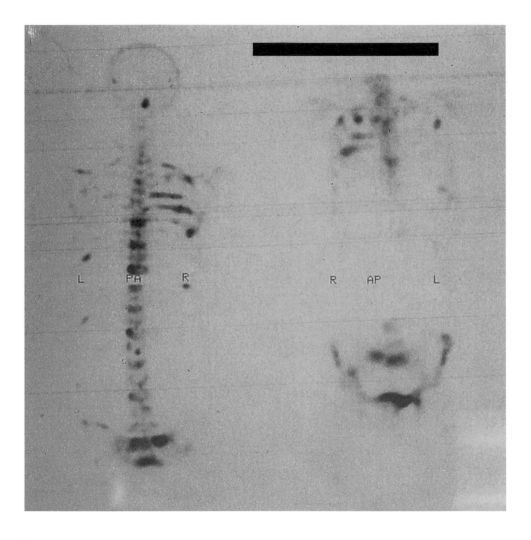

13

A 40-year-old man with diarrhoea describes progressive pain over his lower back and over his buttocks.

What does the X-ray show?
What is the cause of his diarrhoea?

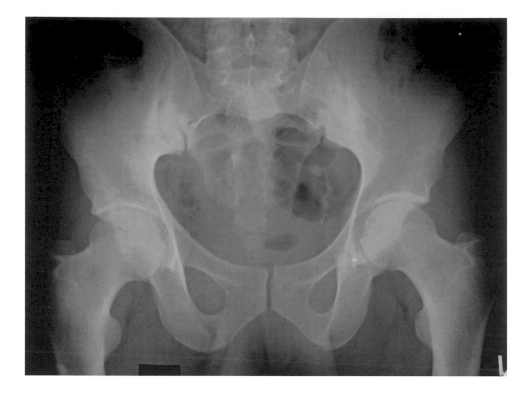

14

A 55-year-old man from Nigeria develops food poisoning after attending a wedding. He develops pain and tenderness over his leg seven days later.

What does the X-ray show?
What is the diagnosis?
What is the likely cause?

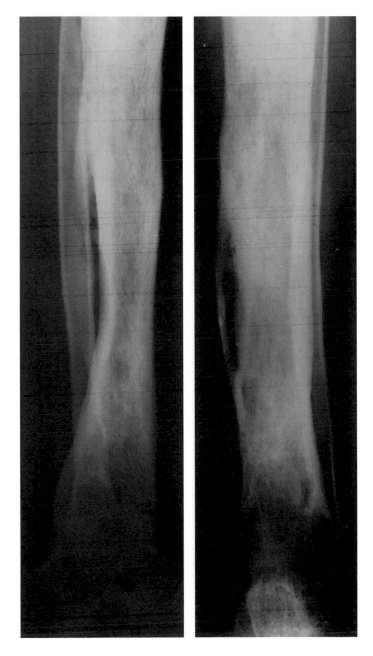

15
A recently married middle-aged man and his wife seek advice when they fail to start a family. On examination, he is tall, with small testes, gynaecomastia and a female distribution of body hair. He complains that he has had back pain for years, and a lumbosacral X-ray is done (*see below and opposite*).

What does it show?
What is the diagnosis?
What condition does this man have?

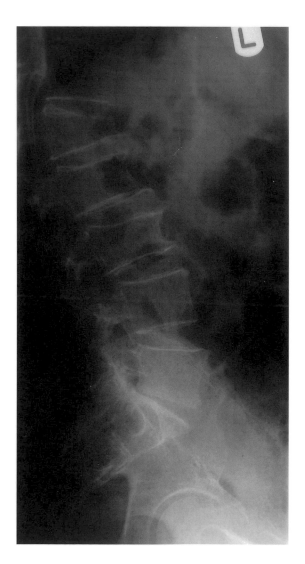

15

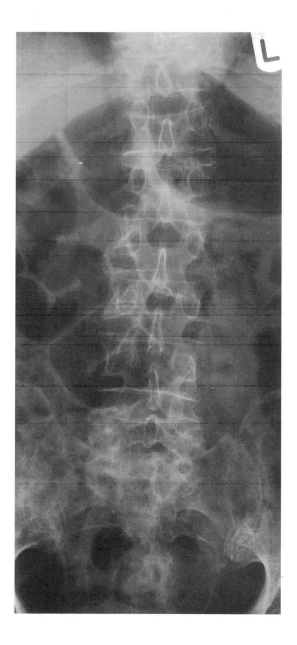

16

These are X-rays of a 65-year-old woman who complains of difficulty in climbing up her stairs.

What do the X-rays show?
What is the diagnosis?
Which tests would you do next?

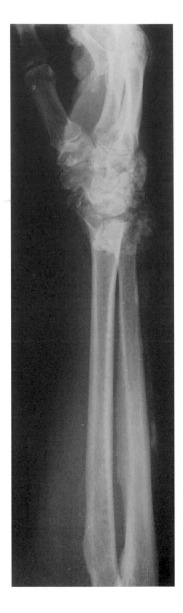
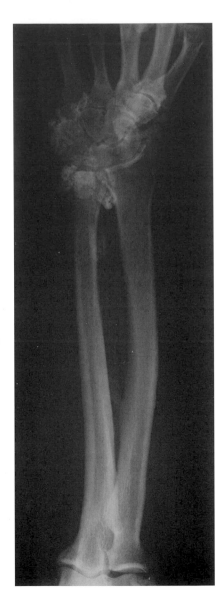

17   This is an X-ray of a show-jumper.

What does it show?
What is the diagnosis?

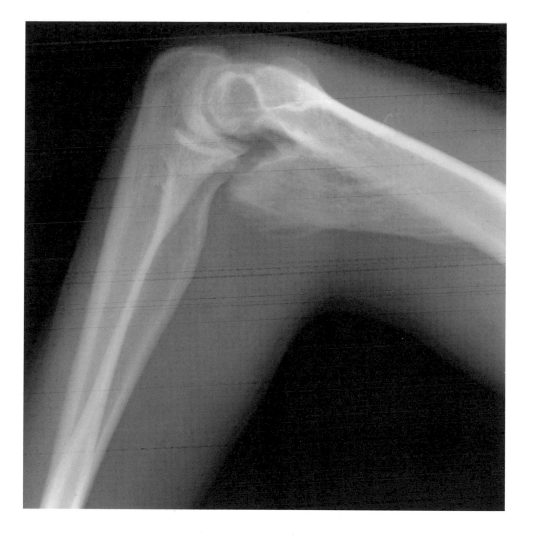

18
These are X-rays of a man complaining of shoulder, knee and ankle pain.

What do they show?
Which test would you do next?

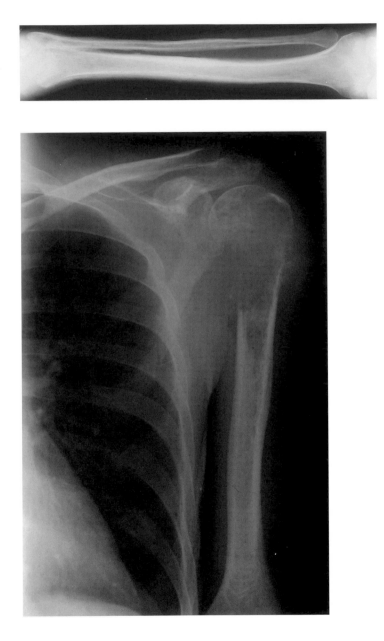

Answers

Cardiology

The CXR shows:
(a) enlargement of the cardiac silhouette;
(b) normal pulmonary vascular markings.

The diagnosis is a pericardial effusion secondary to systemic lupus erythematosus (SLE). This is supported by the history of recurrent miscarriage, thromboembolic disease and epilepsy in a young woman. The features of SLE are protean. The main cardiovascular system (CVS) manifestations are pericardial effusions and Libman–Sachs endocarditis.

Pericardial effusions occur commonly after myocardial infarctions, cardiac surgery, autoimmune disease, viral illness, tuberculosis (TB), malignancy, uraemia and hypothyroidism. Often they are self-limiting, but large effusions can compromise the circulation, particularly if tamponade occurs. Recurrent effusions, which require repeated pericardiocentesis, often require the creation of a surgical window in the pericardium to alleviate the problem. In some cases, constrictive pericarditis may be the long-term sequela of recurrent effusions.

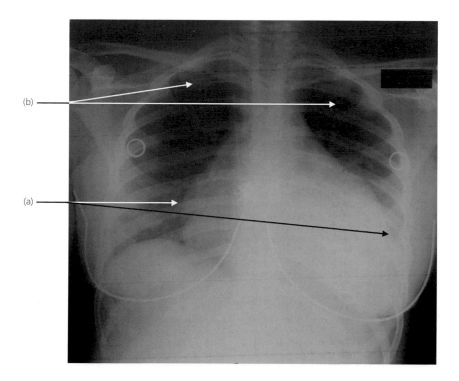

2

This is a pulmonary arteriogram, which shows (see below and opposite):
(a) the normal right pulmonary arterial system;
(b) a saccular dilatation in the left mid-zone, which communicates with;
(c) the left pulmonary artery.

This is a large arteriovenous (AV) malformation arising from the left pulmonary arterial system. This can also be seen with hindsight on the plain film (d). AV malformations may be multiple, and can occur in other organs.

The diagnosis is Osler–Weber–Rendu syndrome (hereditary haemorrhagic telangiectasia), which is an autosomally dominant condition. The telangiectasia arises from focal dilatation of the postcapillary venule. Patients have telangiectasia of the skin and mucosal surfaces, and have insidious or massive blood loss either through the respiratory or gastrointestinal tract. Around 15% of patients have AV malformations, which may lead to a left-to-right shunt if significantly large. Large malformations are treated by embolization. Treatment on the whole is supportive, with iron, blood and anti-fibrinolytics. Treatment with oestrogen analogues may also be of benefit.

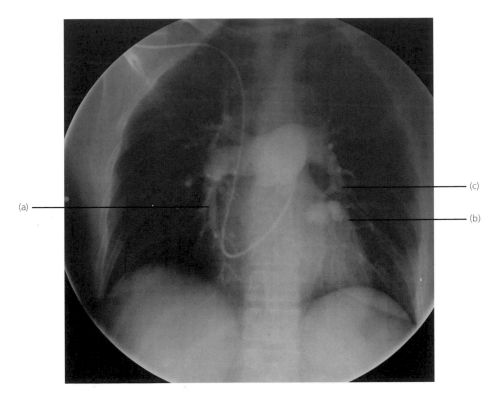

2

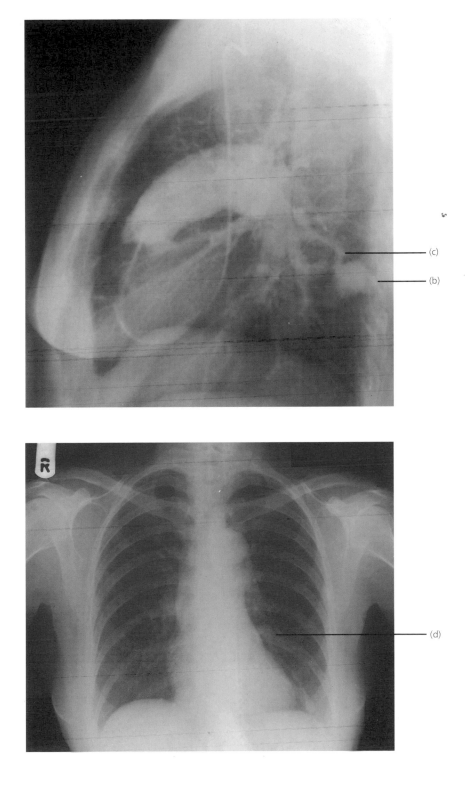

(c)

(b)

(d)

3

This is an underpenetrated A–P CXR and no comments can therefore be made about the heart size. But if we look at the top right corner:
(a) it is clear that the CXR shows dextrocardia, and the X-ray has merely been reversed to make the abnormality less obvious;
(b) the gastric bubble is also under the right hemidiaphragm.

The patient has Kartagener's syndrome. The syndrome includes situs inversus, malformation of the sinuses leading to chronic sinusitis (hence the frontal headaches), bronchiectasis, salpingitis and otitis media. The chance of a male offspring having this condition is probably nil, as males are usually infertile due to immotile sperm. The essential abnormalities are due to the dysmotility of the cilia, caused by defects in the dynein arm. This can be confirmed by nasal biopsy and electron microscopy, or by using tests for ciliary dysmotility such as the nasal saccharin test.

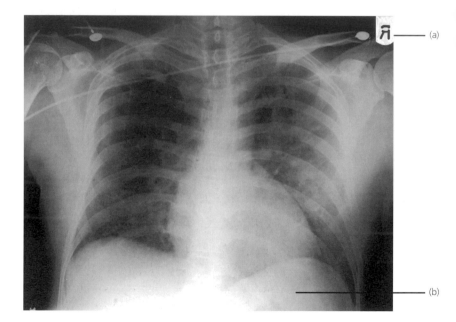

— (a)

— (b)

4

The CT scan of the thorax with contrast shows (see opposite):
(a) a dilated aortic arch;
(b) a contrast-free area in the middle of the arch, which represents a dissection flap in the thoracic aorta.

The CT shows a dissection of a thoracic aneurysm. The patient has developed acute breathlessness due to pulmonary oedema. This is either due to acute aortic incompetence or myocardial infarction. Auscultation of the heart may reveal an early diastolic murmur and a pericardial friction rub.

4

The diagnosis is Marfan's syndrome. This is an autosomal disorder, characterized by abnormalities of collagen. The patients usually have a tall stature, with span greater than height, arachnodactyly, ligament laxity, a high arched palate, upward and lateral dislocation of the lens, kyphosis and pes cavus. Cardiovascular anomalies include aortic regurgitation, mitral valve prolapse, aortic aneurysms and aortic dissection. The gene has variable penetration, and the mortality is highest in those with cardiovascular abnormalities.

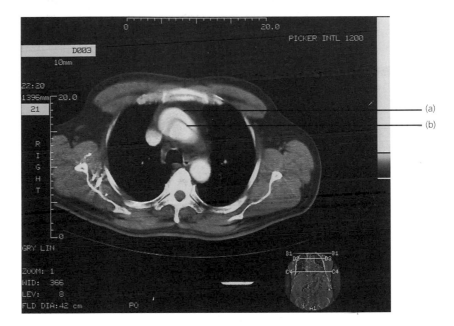

5

The CXR shows (see overleaf top):
(a) rib notching on the undersurface of the ribs;
(b) indentation at the site of narrowing;
(c) pre-stenotic and post-stenotic dilatation which cause the so-called '3 sign' or 'inverted E sign'.

The CXR may also show (see overleaf bottom):
(d) cardiomegaly.

This patient has uncorrected coarctation of the aorta. The visual abnormalities are likely to be due to grade 4 hypertensive retinopathy, which can occur if the coarctation is not corrected. Grades 1 and 2 do not cause visual anomalies, but grade 3 can if the macula is involved. In hypertensive patients, intermittent visual loss may occur due to arterial spasm producing so-called 'visual claudication'.

Coarctation of the aorta, when presenting for the first time in adults, often manifests itself as resistant hypertension. Patients are often well

5

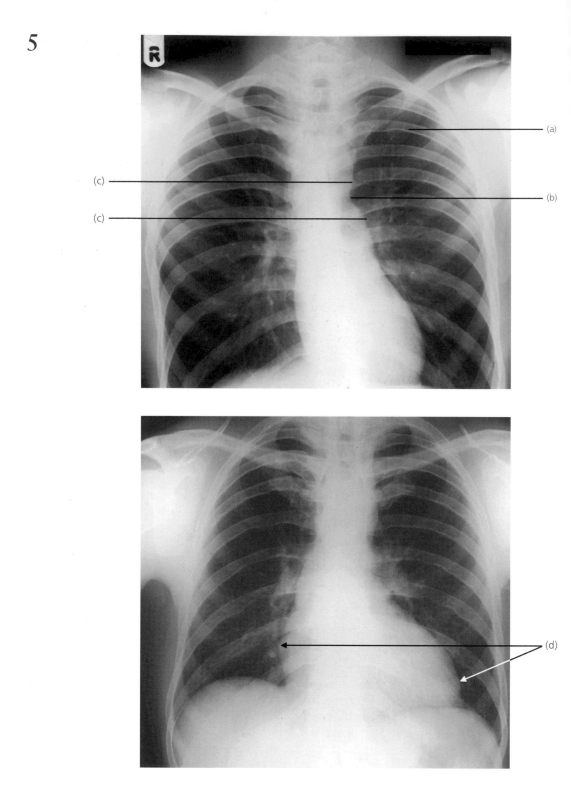

5

developed in their upper bodies and may complain of cold feet, due to poor distal flow. Once the diagnosis is established by cardiac catheterization, the mainstay of treatment is balloon angioplasty. This is usually successful in reducing the gradient, but occasionally surgery is still required. Hypertension is often resistant despite intervention. Mortality remains high, often as a result of strokes.

6

The CXR shows (see below):
(a) a boot-shaped heart (*coeur en sabot*), due to gross enlargement of the right ventricle, which lifts the apex away from the diaphragm;
(b) small pulmonary arteries, leading to
(c) a deep pulmonary bay;
(d) relative oligaemia.

The vascular markings are partially maintained by a supply from the systemic circulation.

Other features that may occur (not shown) are:
(e) a large pulmonary trunk, if pulmonary valvular stenosis is present, as opposed to infundibular stenosis;
(f) rib notching due to enlarged collaterals.

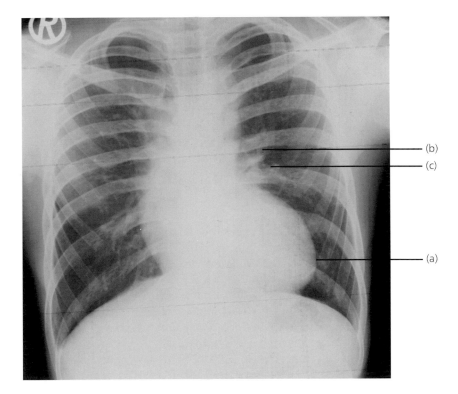

6   The diagnosis is Fallot's tetralogy. The same features may be noted on a chest radiograph of a child (*see below*).

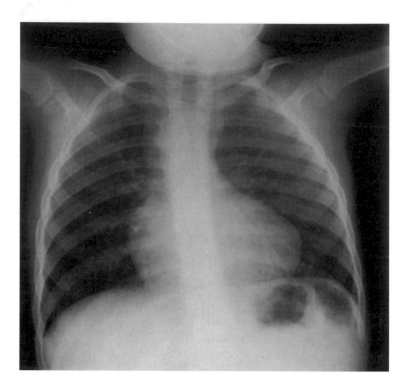

7   *The CXR shows* (*see opposite*):
(a) cardiomegaly;
(b) prominence of the pulmonary trunk;
(c) prominence of the right pulmonary artery;
(d) pulmonary plethora;
(e) small aortic knuckle.

The diagnosis is an atrial septal defect (ASD). There is a left-to-right shunt initially but if the shunt reverses then Eisenmenger's syndrome develops. In this case, the X-ray appearance is similar to that shown here, except that there is peripheral pruning of the pulmonary vasculature due to pulmonary hypertension. The pulmonary plethora may also diminish after transcatheter or surgical closure. Transcatheter closure is suitable for secundum ASD defects that have a rim sufficiently large for the device to be attached.

The stroke is likely to have been caused by a paradoxical embolus from a pelvic vein or deep vein thrombus in the peripartum period.

7

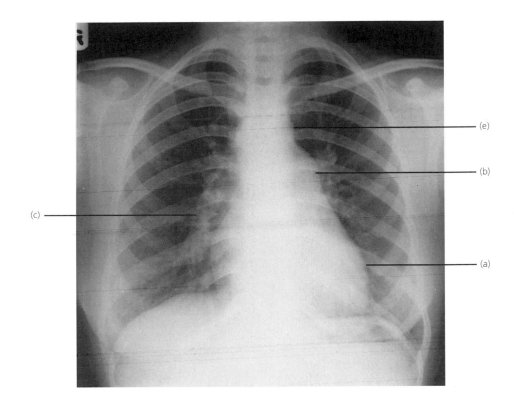

(e)

(b)

(c)

(a)

8

The CXR shows (see overleaf top and bottom):
(a) pericardial calcification (shown by arrowheads).

The likely diagnosis, in the absence of other radiological anomalies, is constrictive pericarditis. Almost half of these patients have some degree of pericardial calcification. Occasionally, there may be clues to the aetiology, e.g. the presence of calcification or fibrosis in the apices suggesting a tuberculous origin.

Cardiac catheterization showing elevated left atrium (LA) and right atrium (RA) pressures and equalization of diastolic pressures in the left and right heart would support the diagnosis.

The clinical features are mainly of right-heart failure with severe ascites and hepatosplenomegaly. Other signs include an elevated JVP which rises on inspiration (Kusmal's sign), pulsus paradoxus and a loud third heart sound (pericardial knock).

Constrictive pericarditis develops insidiously, and may be secondary to any cause of acute pericarditis. It is more common when the pericardial fluid is haemorrhagic or purulent, e.g. malignant disease or TB. Treatment is by surgical resection of the pericardium.

8

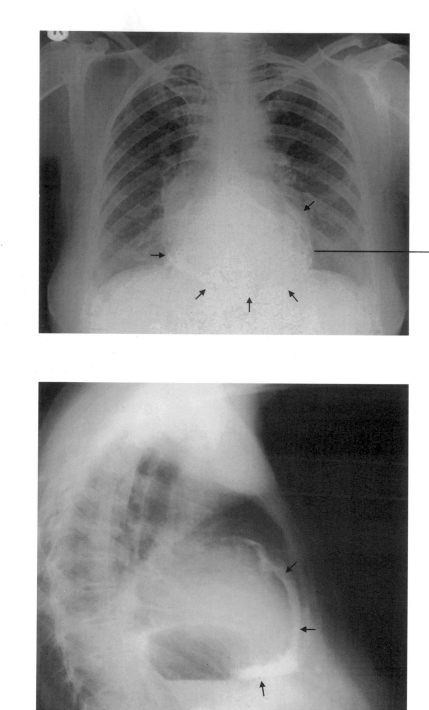

(a)

9

The CXR shows (see below):
(a) cardiomegaly;
(b) a double heart shadow;
(c) prominence of the pulmonary trunk;
(d) upper lobe diversion;
(e) pulmonary ossification;
(f) enlarged left atrial appendage;
(g) calcification of the mitral valve.

The lateral X-ray shows (see overleaf):
(h) calcification of the mitral valve;
(i) left atrial enlargement.

The diagnosis is mitral stenosis.

The haemoptysis is secondary to pulmonary venous hypertension and hence capillary leakage. Patients present with progressive breathlessness or haemoptysis. Sudden deterioration in their cardiac status usually heralds the onset of atrial fibrillation (AF). Severe symptomatic cases are treated with mitral balloon valvuloplasty, which not only increases the mitral valve area, but helps to maintain sinus rhythm. Suitable patients are those in whom there is little or no mitral regurgitation (MR), an intact subvalvular apparatus and an absence of thrombus. Those not suitable may still be candidates for valve repair, and the rest may require valve replacement.

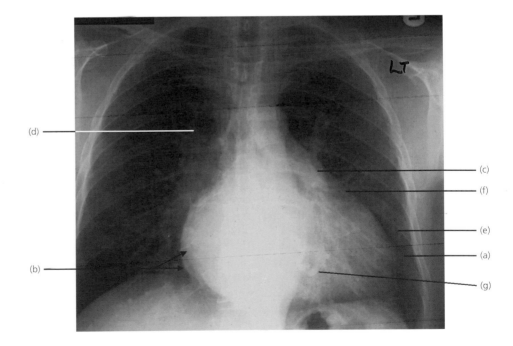

9

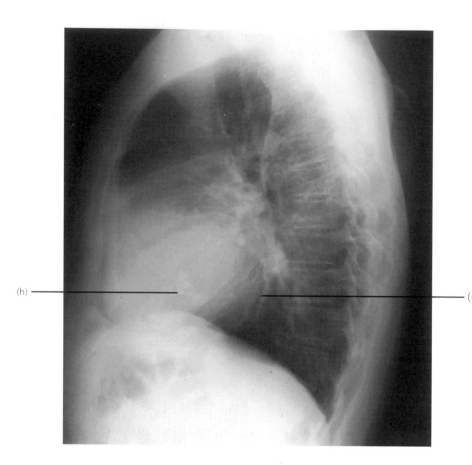

(h) ————————————————   ———————————— (i)

10

The MRI scan shows narrowing and thickening of the walls of (see opposite):
(a) the right subclavian artery;
(b) the right internal carotid artery;
(c) the left internal carotid artery;

Rarely, the aortic arch may show:
(d) aneurysmal dilatation (not shown).

The diagnosis is Takayasu's disease. This is more common in women and in Japanese people. It presents between 20 and 40 years of age. Patients complain of fever, malaise, fatigue and arthralgia. Cardiovascular symptoms include dyspnoea and claudication. The disease is often only diagnosed during the occlusive phase. Examination reveals absent pulses, bruits and hypertension. Hypertension occurs as a result of an 'acquired' coarctation of the aorta, or through involvement of the renal arteries. Other tests used to ascertain the diagnosis include an aortogram, a perfusion scan and a digital subtraction angiogram.

10   Corticosteroids and anticoagulation therapy may result in a return of the arterial pulses, with surgery being indicated for acute ischaemia or intractable hypertension.

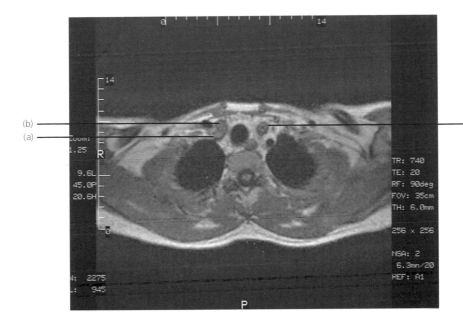

11   *The left ventricle (LV) angiogram shows (see overleaf top):*
(a) a dilated left ventricle;
(b) a filling defect at the apex.

This is a thrombus in the left ventricle (LV), which has intermittently been embolizing and giving rise to transient ischaemic attacks (TIAs). The patient should receive full anticoagulation treatment and an echocardiogram should be performed at a later date to assess whether the thrombus has resolved.

Left ventricular thrombus commonly occurs adjacent to hypokinetic or akinetic segments. Anticoagulation should be considered in patients with impaired left ventricular function in the presence of atrial fibrillation, or if an aneurysm is present.

A typical example of an LV aneurysm is shown (*see overleaf bottom*). It shows:
(c) cardiomegaly;
(d) bulge on the left heart border.

In cases of intractable heart failure aneurysmectomy should be considered.

11

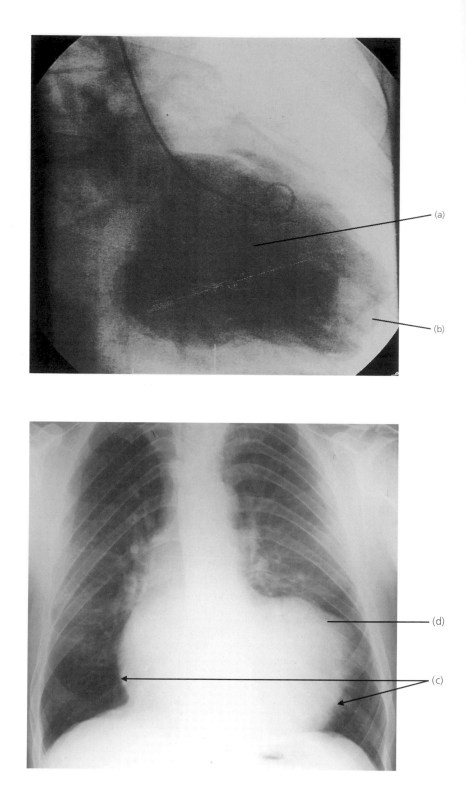

12

The CXR shows (see below):
(a) cardiomegaly;
(b) double heart shadow;
(c) prominent pulmonary trunk;
(d) upper lobe diversion;
(e) pulmonary ossification;
(f) a thoracotomy scar;
(g) pericardial calcification.

Note that the left atrial appendage is not as enlarged as in the case shown in Question 9, and therefore previous mitral valve surgery is likely, as the LA appendage is usually removed at operation. This patient has undergone valve surgery in the past. The sternal wires are not easily seen in the P–A view. The thoracotomy suggests that she has also had mitral valvotomy prior to valve replacement.

The lateral CXR shows (see overleaf top):
(h) the mitral valve prosthesis;
(i) the tricuspid valve prosthesis;
(j) an enlarged left atrium.

Atria as large as these may give rise to dysphagia, and a barium swallow can be used to demonstrate this (*see overleaf bottom*). The shortness of breath in this case may be due to regurgitation from the valve prosthesis, or may be the development of atrial fibrillation.

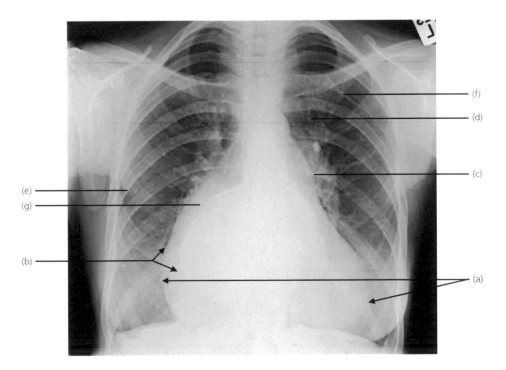

12

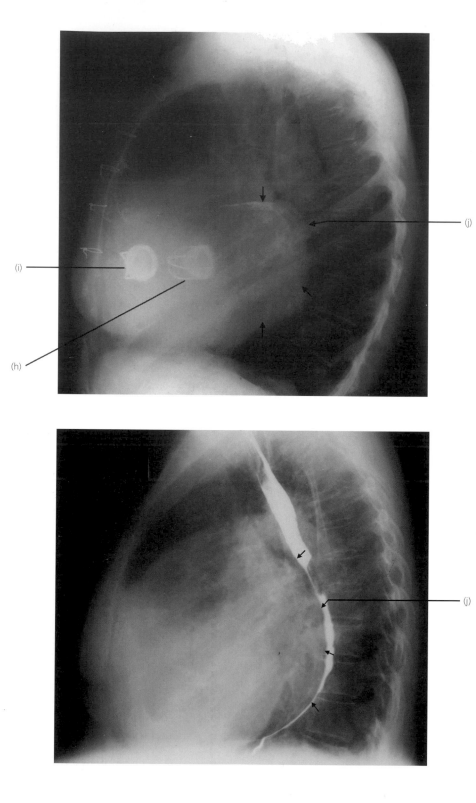

13 *The plain abdominal X-ray shows*:
(a) a dilated abdominal aorta (shown by arrowheads);
(b) calcification of the walls of the aorta.

The diagnosis is aneurysm of the abdominal aorta. These aneurysms usually occur below the level of the renal arteries, but around 5% are suprarenal. Although asymptomatic in the majority of cases, they may give rise to distal vascular embolization. Emergency surgery for rupture of the aneurysm is associated with a high mortality, but elective repair carries a risk of around 5%. This is usually undertaken for aneurysms greater than 5 cm in diameter (where there is a favourable risk–benefit ratio), or 4–5 cm if there are no other cardiovascular risk factors present. Six-monthly screening using ultrasonography is recommended. There may be a benefit from beta blockade, as it is postulated that this reduces the rate of expansion of the aneurysm. Currently, transfemoral endovascular repair is being undertaken with increasing success in high-risk cases.

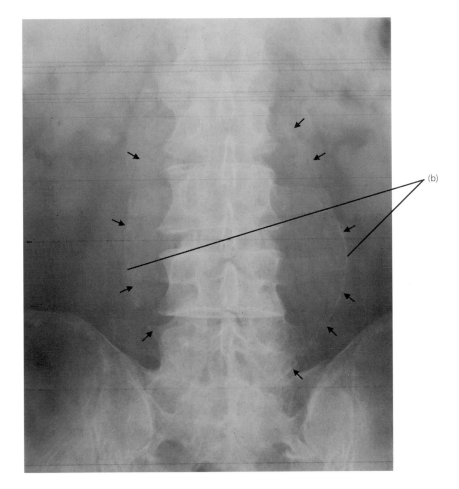

(b)

14   *This is a stress thallium scan (see facing plate).* The patient undergoes chemical and handgrip testing, followed by the injection of thallium. A gamma camera takes pictures of the stressed heart, and later of the heart in a resting state after a second injection of thallium.

(a) The first picture (the stress image) shows a clear anterior perfusion defect, seen as a dark blue area on the 'bull's-eye image'.
(b) The normal resting perfusion scan shows no perfusion defects.

This shows reversible ischaemia in the left anterior descending artery territory. An infarct would show up as a fixed perfusion defect in both images.

Shortness of breath is a manifestation of ischaemia, although it is uncommon by itself. The patient should therefore have coronary angiography and possibly balloon angioplasty. Coronary risk factors such as smoking, cholesterol, high-density lipoproteins (HDLs), blood pressure and weight should be aggressively treated in a man of this age. The greatest impact on mortality in this case will be achieved through cessation of smoking and lipid reduction.

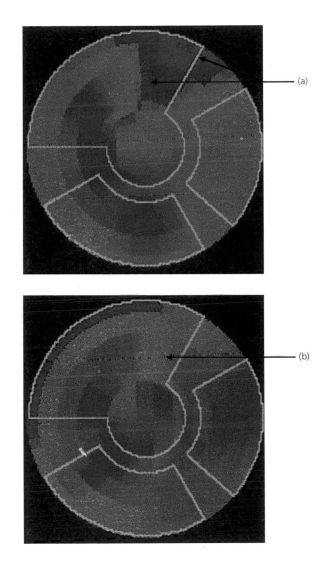

(a)

(b)

Endocrinology

1

The skull X-rays show (see below and overleaf top):
(a) enlargement of the pituitary fossa;
(b) prominence of the frontal and zygomatic bones;
(c) prominence of the supraorbital ridge;
(d) destruction of the anterior and posterior clinoid process;
(e) prognathism;
(f) wide separation of the teeth.
(g) In addition, a 'double floor' of the sella may be seen in less severe cases (not shown).

The diagnosis is acromegaly. Excessive secretion of growth hormone after epiphyseal fusion has occurred, which leads to the typical appearance shown. Visceromegaly also occurs, with enlargement of the liver, spleen and heart. Patients usually die from cardiovascular complications such as heart failure and myocardial infarction. Hypertension and stroke are also common.

The diagnosis can be confirmed by the failure of suppression of growth hormone during a 75-g oral glucose tolerance test (OGTT). Treatment is surgical, via a trans-sphenoidal or frontal approach, with

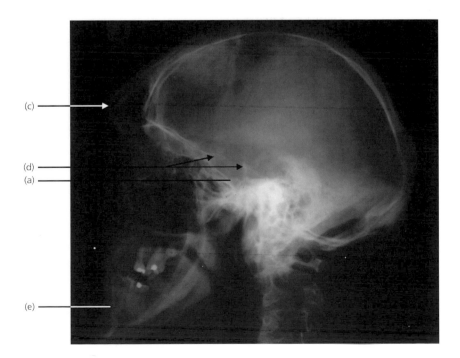

1

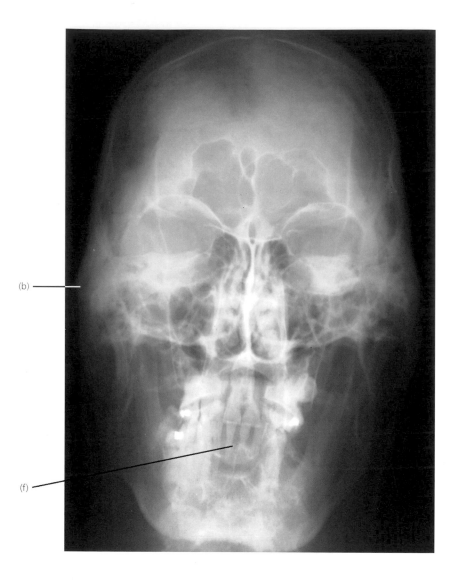

(b)

(f)

or without adjuvant radiotherapy. About 75% of patients respond to bromocriptine. Somatostatin analogues such as octreotide may also be given to reduce the effects of insulin-like growth factor I (IGF-I), which in turn can be used as a marker of disease activity.

2

The X-ray shows (see opposite top):
(a) spade-like hand;
(b) tufting of the terminal phalanges;
(c) an increase in joint space, due to cartilage overgrowth;
(d) an increase in the amount of soft tissue.

The X-ray (*see opposite bottom*) shows the typical appearance of the feet in this condition. The diagnosis is acromegaly.

2

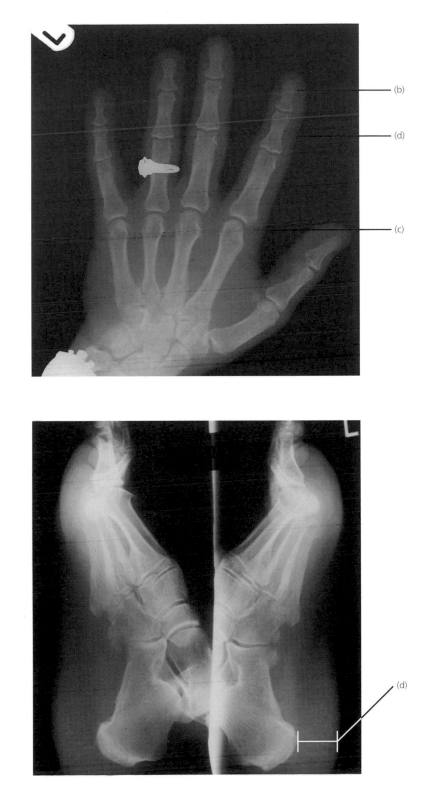

3

This X-ray of the thoracolumbar spine shows:
(a) new bone formation at the anterior margins of the vertebrae;
(b) an increase in the A–P diameter of the vertebral bodies.
(c) Fistular scalloping and prominent marginal osteophyte formation are also characteristic.

The diagnosis is acromegaly.
    The tingling in the hands is due to soft tissue compression of the median nerve. This is causing carpal tunnel syndrome.

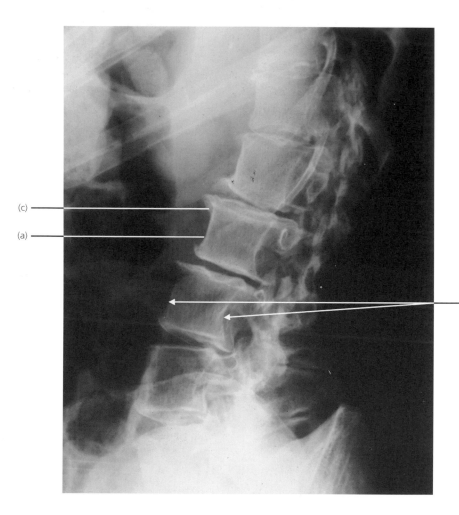

4

The CT scan of the abdomen shows (see below and overleaf):
(a) a large adrenal mass in the medulla. This is a phaeochromocytoma.

The diagnosis is multiple endocrine neoplasia (MEN) type 2b. This particular syndrome is characterized by a marfanoid habitus (skeletal deformity, but no eye or cardiovascular system complications), phaeochromocytoma (70% are bilateral), medullary carcinoma of the thyroid, and parathyroid hyperplasia (60%). Mandatory biochemical tests are 24-hour urinary metanephrines or catecholamines for phaeochromocytoma, calcitonin for medullary cancer of the thyroid and Ca, PO_4 and parathyroid hormone (PTH) for hyperparathyroidism.

Neurofibromas are often present, with 5% being mucosal. Treatment is by surgery with perioperative alpha and beta blockade. Diabetes is often secondary to excess catecholamine secretion, and normoglycaemia may return after surgery.

(a) ——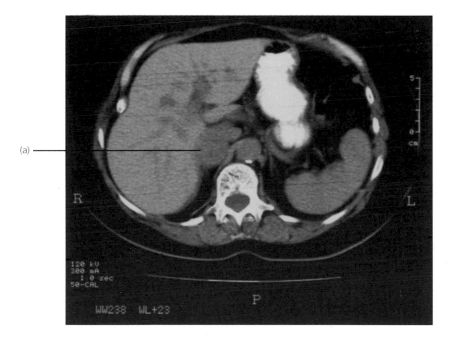

4

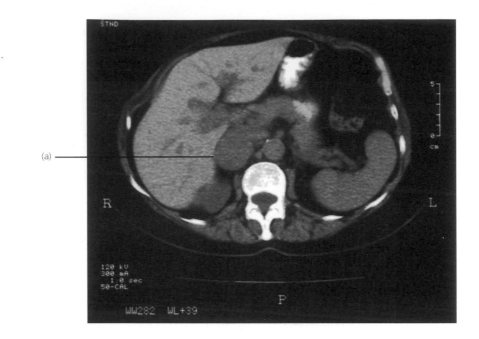

(a)

5

The chest X-ray shows (see opposite):
(a) lung fibrosis.

She has presented in Addisonian crisis. The aetiology of the adrenal failure is tuberculosis, which is the commonest cause of this condition in developing countries. An abdominal X-ray might show adrenal gland calcification. In developed countries, autoimmune disease is the main cause, and may be associated with multiple autoimmune endocrinopathy, such as type 1 diabetes mellitus, primary hypoparathyroidism, pernicious anaemia, vitiligo, autoimmune thyroid disease and premature ovarian failure in women.

In addition to the symptoms described, patients will have increased pigmentation inside the buccal cavity, in skin creases and also extensor surfaces. Biochemical tests would confirm a low Na, high K and low glucose. The basal level of cortisol is low and fails to respond to tetracosactrin (Synacthen). Long-term therapy involves treatment with hydrocortisone and fludrocortisone, with doses of hydrocortisone being increased during times of physiological stress, e.g. intercurrent bacterial infection.

5

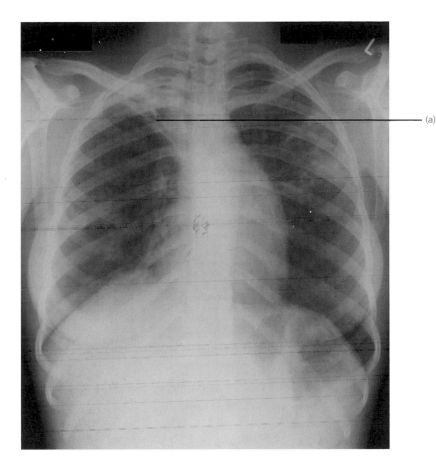

———————— (a)

6

The MRI scan shows (see overleaf):
(a) a pituitary tumour, with a typical sloping floor;
(b) with suprasellar extension;
(c) infiltration of the cavernous sinus on the left (cf. the right side);
(d) a bright area within the tumour, which is due to infarction
(also seen in patients on bromocriptine treatment).

This is a pituitary macroadenoma. The next scan (*see p. 205 top*) shows distortion and displacement of the optic chiasm (e).

The combination of galactorrhoea and a pituitary tumour makes the diagnosis of prolactinoma most likely. This can be confirmed by the presence of a serum prolactin of >4000 IU. There is a sixth nerve palsy due to infiltration of the cavernous sinus by the tumour. The sixth nerve lies more medially compared to cranial nerves III and IV, and is therefore the first to be affected.

Prolactinoma is the commonest type of pituitary tumour, and presents with symptoms of amenorrhoea or galactorrhoea in women, or impo-

6

tence, headache and diplopia in men. Once the diagnosis is confirmed, the treatment is by dopaminergic agents such as bromocriptine, even in cases of pituitary macroadenoma. Measurements of visual fields are essential, and an increase in visual field loss (upper quadrantanopia and then bitemporal hemianopia) despite medical therapy is an indication for urgent surgery, with or without adjunctive radiotherapy. Counselling in women is essential, as prolactinomas may enlarge during pregnancy and the experience with the newer dopamine agonists (cabergoline and quinagolide) is insufficient to be certain of their safety during pregnancy. There is greater experience during pregnancy with bromocriptine itself, but even this agent is usually only considered for possible use in pregnancy if the pituitary is shown to be enlarging. Regular measurements of visual fields are essential here. Regular measurements of visual fields are essential here.

The next MRI scan (*see opposite bottom*) shows a pituitary microadenoma (f) for comparison with the above. Note that there is no suprasellar extension (g) and that the optic chiasm is intact (h). Pituitary stalk compression by any pituitary macroadenoma (i.e., even if not a prolactinoma) can lead to an increase in prolactin by interfering with the normal dopamine supression of prolactin secreting cells. In this situation the prolactin level is usually <4000 IU.

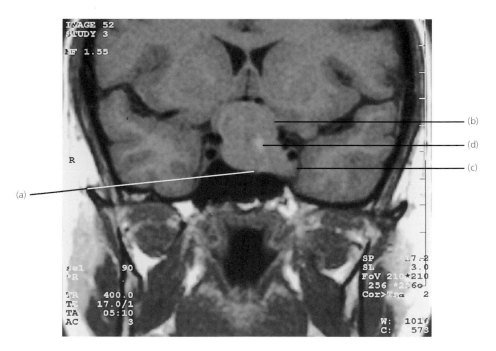

6

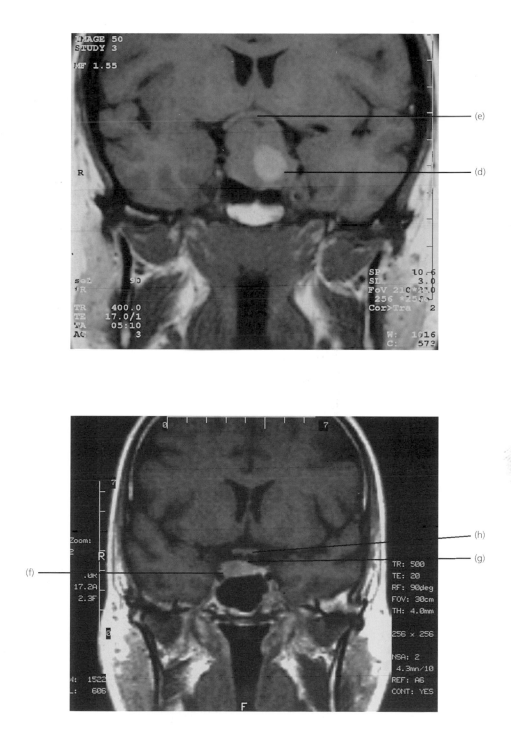

7   *The skull X-ray shows (see top below):*
(a) a typical ground-glass (granular) appearance;
(b) cyst formation.

This appearance is often referred to as a 'pepper-pot skull'.

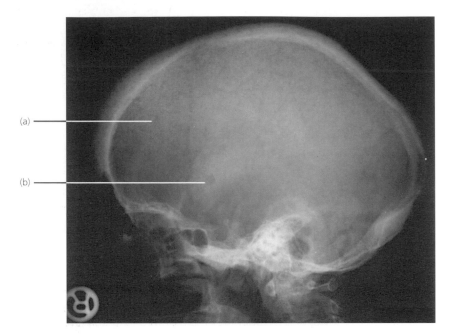

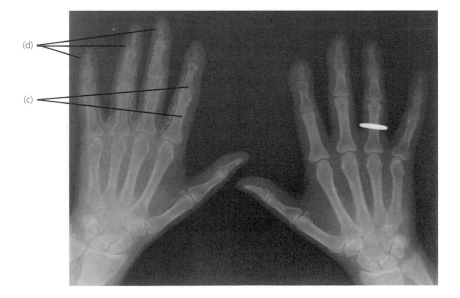

7

The radiographs of the hands show (see opposite below):
(c) subperiosteal erosions along the cortical surfaces of the middle and distal phalanges;
(d) gross resorption of the distal phalanges.

The diagnosis is hyperparathyroidism. This can be diagnosed by confirming an elevated PTH in the presence of an increased serum calcium and a low phosphate. Hypercalcaemia leads to vomiting. The formation of renal stones leads to loin pain, and tubular damage then leads to polyuria. Other presentations are with peptic ulcers and pancreatitis.

Hypercalcaemia should be treated by rehydration and osteoclast inhibitors, such as pamidronate. Curative treatment is by parathyroidectomy.

8

The X-ray shows (see below):
(a) brachydactyly, i.e. shortening of the fingers;
(b) it is especially pronounced in the fourth and fifth metacarpals.

The diagnosis is pseudohypoparathyroidism. Those affected have characteristic somatic features, such as short stature, mental retardation, round facies, short necks and abnormal dentition. There is a low serum calcium with an appropriately elevated PTH level. This is thought to be due to an abnormality of the PTH receptor. Occasionally, X-rays show osteitis fibrosa, indicating skeletal sensitivity to PTH hormone.

There is also a condition known as pseudopseudohypoparathyroidism, in which patients have the somatic features described above,

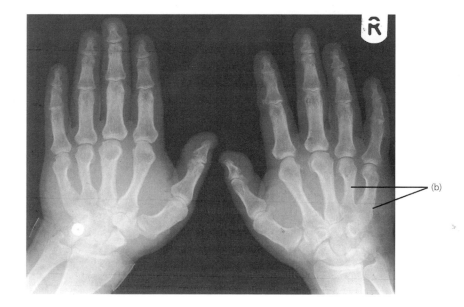

8

but normal Ca, PO_4 and PTH. These patients are often close relations of people with pseudohypoparathyroidism. Other features in this group are the presence of cataracts at an early age.

9

This is a ^{99m}Tc scan, which shows:
(a) multiple areas of increased uptake in the thyroid gland;
(b) the rest of the thyroid gland does not take up the isotope (cold spots).

The diagnosis is toxic multinodular goitre of the thyroid gland. The patient may have lid lag. This is a manifestation of thyrotoxicosis. Exophthalmos is a manifestation of Graves' disease and not raised free T_4 alone.

Thyrotoxicosis is common, and has a prevalence of around 2%, being five times more common in women. In the elderly it presents insidiously, with weight loss, atrial fibrillation (50%) and congestive cardiac failure. Eye signs are uncommon, in contrast to the younger population, in which there are a number of manifestations of thyroid disease (Graves' disease). In the younger group, cardiovascular system (CVS) signs are less common, and the thyroid disease is due to immunoglobulin G (IgG) autoantibodies stimulating the thyroid-stimulating hormone (TSH) receptor. In the elderly, toxic multinodular goitre and toxic adenoma in a goitre make up a larger proportion of the cases.

Treatment is medical initially with carbimazole or propylthiouracil, but large goitres may not remit on medical therapy. Toxic adenoma or a toxic multinodular goitre may be treated when euthyroid by subtotal

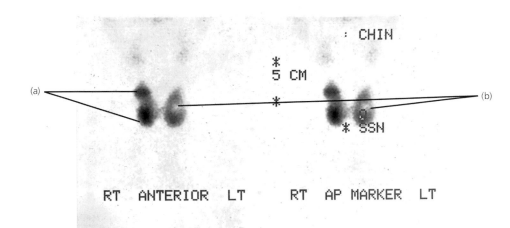

9 thyroidectomy, or radioiodine (^{131}I) treatment. In cases in which there is no adenoma, radioiodine is the treatment of choice, rendering 75% of patients euthyroid in the short term. There is a high incidence of hypothyroidism over the subsequent 20 years, however. Patients undergoing subtotal thyroidectomy should stop antithyroid drugs 10–14 days prior to surgery. Potassium iodide is given in the interim to reduce the vascularity of the gland.

10 *The MRI scan shows (see below):*
(a) a craniopharyngioma with suprasellar extension;
(b) destruction of the pituitary;
(c) there also appears to be compression of the optic chiasm.

The patient is bumping into objects because of a bitemporal hemianopia. The patient was treated surgically, and postoperative hydrocephalus is likely to have occurred, as the second X-ray shows (*see overleaf*):
(d) insertion of a ventriculoperitoneal shunt.

Craniopharyngioma presents insidiously in children or in the elderly with panhypopituitarism. Other presentations are with visual field loss (lower bitemporal quadrantanopia, which progresses to bitemporal hemianopia), hydrocephalus due to compression of the third ventricle,

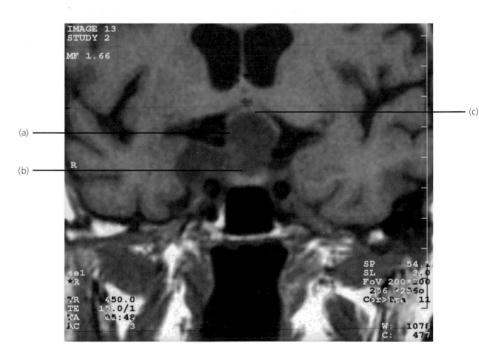

10

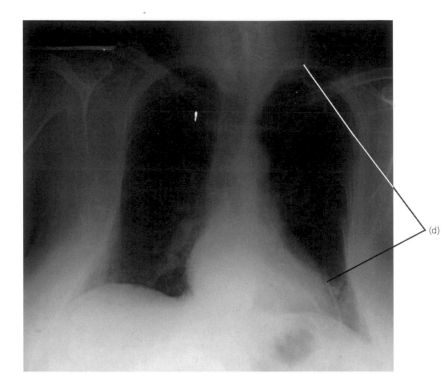

or incidentally as calcification on a lateral skull X-ray (50% of the lesions are calcified). Treatment is surgical via the trans-sphenoidal or transfrontal route, followed by hormone replacement therapy with hydrocortisone, fludrocortisone and thyroxine. Men may also need testosterone, and premenopausal women may require oestrogen.

11

These are X-rays of the thoracic inlet. They show (see opposite top and bottom):
(a) deviation of the trachea (shown by arrowheads);
(b) flecks of calcification around the trachea;
(c) soft tissue swelling in the neck (in the region of the thyroid gland).

The diagnosis is thoracic inlet syndrome secondary to a thyroid mass.

Serum T_4 and TSH and thyroid autoantibody tests should be carried out to assess thyroid status and to look for evidence of autoimmune thyroid disease. Other investigations include ultrasound scan of the thyroid to determine whether the mass is cystic or solid, and fine-needle aspiration (FNA) for cytology.

11

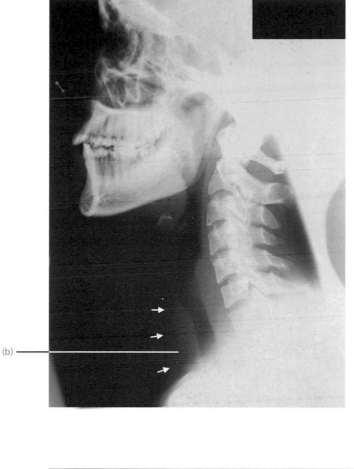

(b)

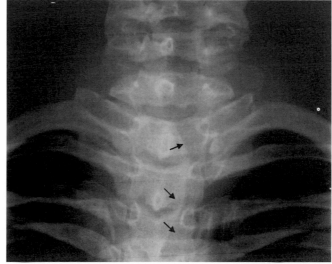

12   *This is a ⁹⁹ᵐTc methoxyisobutylisonitrile (MIBI) subtraction scan:*
(a) MIBI is taken up by the thyroid gland and the parathyroid gland;
(b) Tc is taken up by the thyroid gland alone;
(c) digital subtraction confirms a parathyroid adenoma.

The renal failure is secondary to hypercalcaemia. Treatment is by parathyroidectomy.

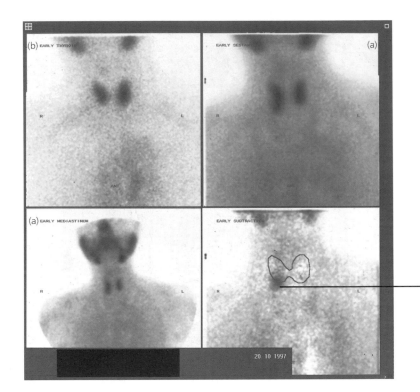

13   *The radiograph shows (see opposite):*
(a) a mass in the region of the thoracic inlet.

This is a retrosternal goitre. The next step would be to establish the patient's thyroid status (see Question 9).

13

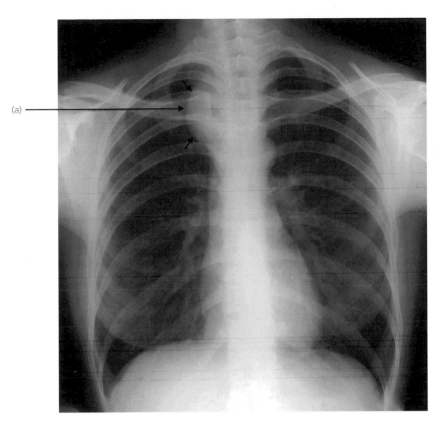

(a)

Gastroenterology

1

The barium swallow shows (see below and opposite):
(a) an oesophageal web at the level of D 4.

This is Paterson–Brown Kelly or Plummer–Vinson syndrome. It is caused by submucosal inflammation, principally in the postcricoid region, producing a web or stenosis. Patients present with dysphagia or symptoms of anaemia. Classically, patients have features of chronic iron deficiency such as koilonychia or atrophic glossitis. Women are affected more commonly than men. This condition is a premalignant finding.

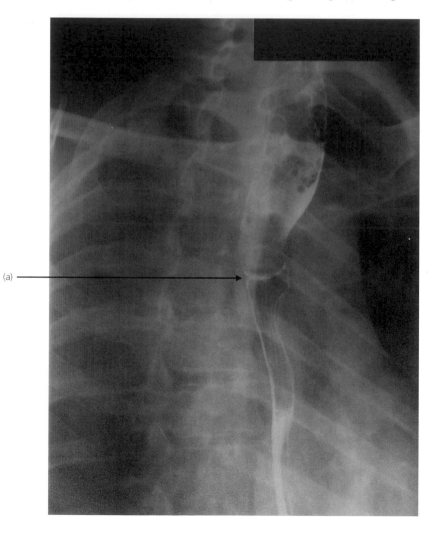

(a)

1

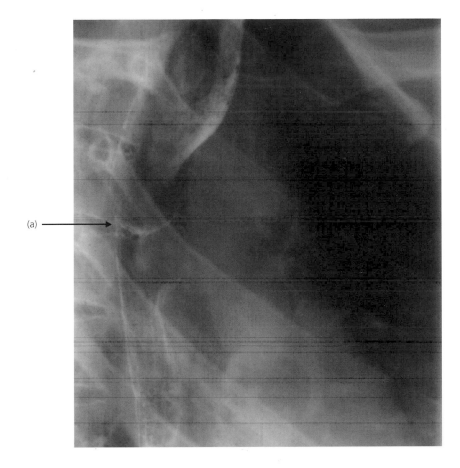

(a) →

2

The plain abdominal X-ray shows (see overleaf top):
(a) small-bowel intestinal obstruction.

The later barium study shows (see overleaf bottom):
(b) a small-bowel polyp.

This is Peutz–Jeghers syndrome, an autosomal dominant condition in which gastrointestinal tract hamartomatous polyps are associated with mucocutaneous pigmentation of the lips, hands and feet.

The major complications are anaemia due to excessive bleeding, intussusception, intestinal obstruction and malignant transformation. Malignant transformation is rare, except in the stomach and duodenum. Small-intestinal resection is advised for polyps >1 cm in size and in cases of intussusception.

2

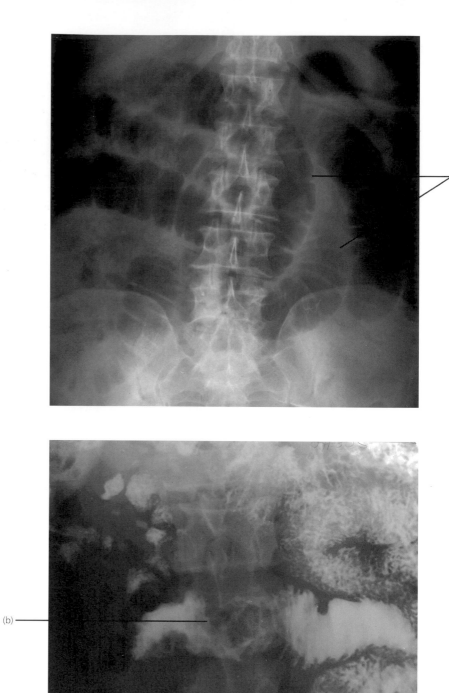

3

The endoscopic retrograde cholangiopancreatogram (ERCP) shows:
(a) dilatation of the biliary tree;
(b) stricturing of the biliary tree.

The diagnosis is primary sclerosing cholangitis. This is a rare but serious complication of inflammatory bowel disease, and its progression leads to secondary biliary cirrhosis with portal hypertension.

Other complications of ulcerative colitis (UC) are fatty changes in the liver, pericholangitis, cholangiocarcinoma, cancer of the gallbladder and cirrhosis. Panproctocolectomy may arrest the progression of the cirrhosis. Other complications associated with ulcerative colitis are gallstones, renal stones (note that calculi more common in Crohn's disease), uveitis, seronegative arthropathy, pyoderma gangrenosum and erythema nodosum.

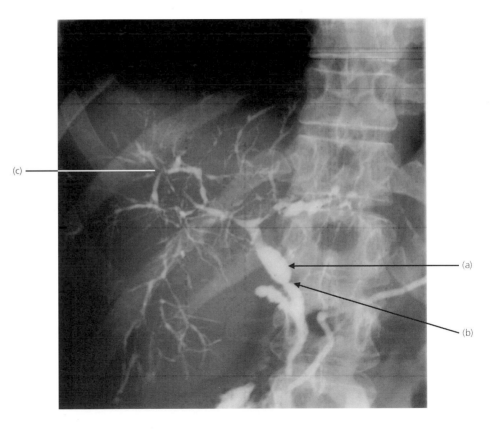

4

The barium studies show (see below and opposite top):
(a) thickening of the valvulae conniventes;
(b) areas of dilatation and narrowing that alternate with normal mucosa, i.e. skip lesions;
(c) a narrow stricture at the distal end of the terminal ileum, which represents the string sign (of Kantor).

These radiological signs are pathognomonic of Crohn's disease. Other radiological abnormalities include (not shown):
(d) cobblestoning;
(e) fissuring and thinning of the walls.

A plain AXR (see opposite bottom) may be useful in active disease, as it may show:
(f) mucosal oedema ('thumb-printing');
(g) loss of haustrations (colonic Crohn's);
(h) a mass in the right iliac fossa (not shown);
(i) sacroilitis

The patient is anaemic, with a macrocytosis. In the context of small-bowel Crohn's disease, this could be due to malabsorption of vitamin B_{12} due to a terminal ileitis or folate malabsorption in the upper small intestine. The former is more likely, and can be confirmed by serum B_{12} and folate tests. Without the above radiological signs, the next step would be a Dicopac test.

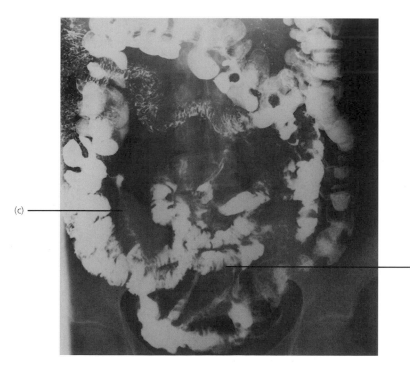

4

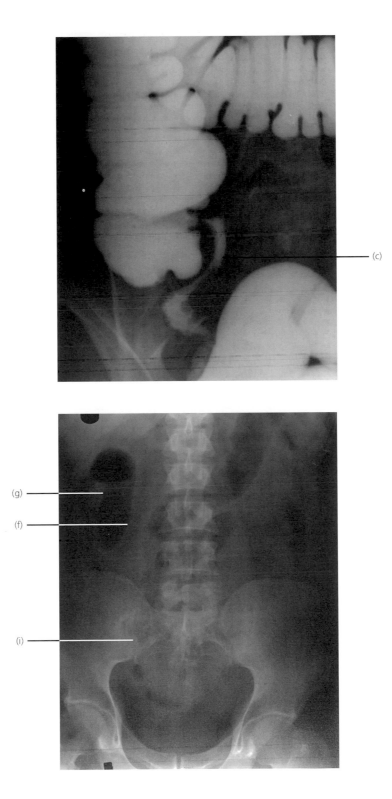

5

The CXR shows:
(a) a fluid level behind the heart;
(b) inflammatory changes at the base of the right lung.

This is due to a hiatus hernia, which has resulted in recurrent episodes of aspiration pneumonia. A hiatus hernia may occur by the stomach pushing up besides the oesophagus (paraoesophageal) or, in 80% of cases, it may herniate directly, leading to the so-called sliding hiatus hernia. This condition is commonest in multiparous women and in the obese. Patients complain of a fullness in the chest, shortness of breath (SOB) and chest pain. Lying flat or bending over leads to reflux, as the normal sphincter mechanism of the gastro-oesophageal junction becomes incompetent. Aspiration leads to a chemical pneumonitis of the right lower lobe in the erect patient, or the posterior segment of the right upper lobe in the supine patient. Patients are advised to sleep upright, and proton-pump inhibitors are used to reduce the oesophagitis. Surgery (Nissen fundoplication) is considered in severe cases.

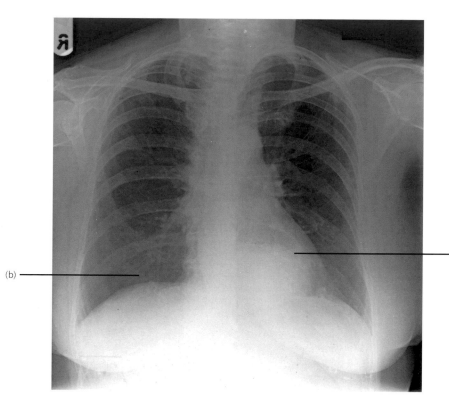

(b)

(a)

6

The double-contrast barium enema shows (see below):
(a) loss of the normal haustral patterns;
(b) a smooth tubular appearance of the colon;
(c) discrete ulcers;
(d) so-called 'pseudopolyps', which represent mucosal oedema and appear as filling defects.

The above appearance is continuous throughout the colon.

A single-contrast barium study in another patient (*see overleaf top*) shows:
(e) 'tramline appearance' in ulcerative colitis.

This represents the presence of barium in the deep mucosal ulcers, and is the typical appearance of ulcerative colitis. Acute complications are massive haemorrhage, perforation and toxic dilatation (f) (*see overleaf bottom*). There is an increased risk of colonic cancer after 10 years. Other complications are listed in Question 3 (*see p. 217*).

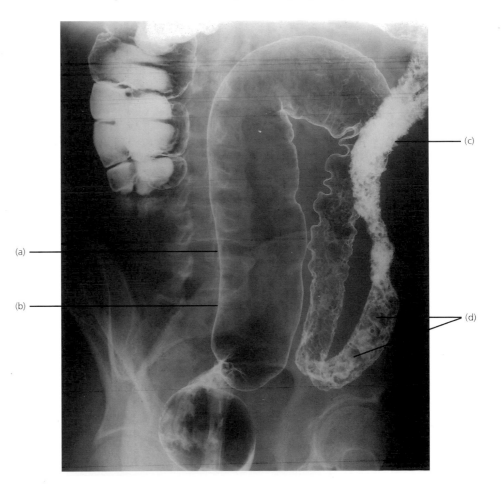

6

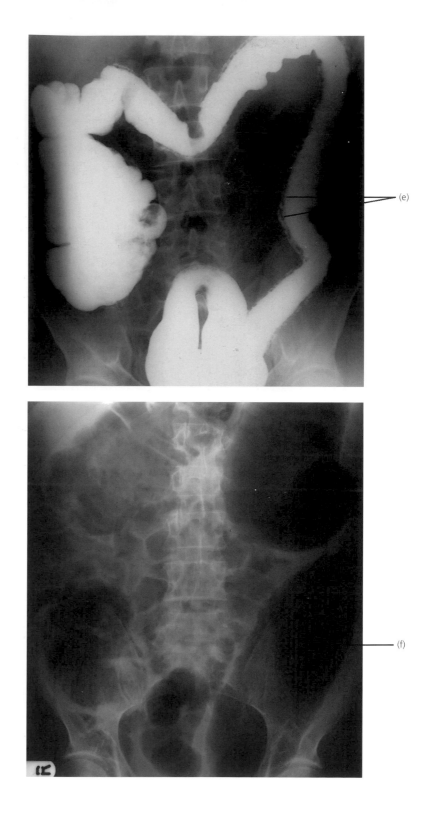

(e)

(f)

7

The abdominal X-ray shows:
(a) calcification in the region of the pancreas, indicating chronic pancreatitis (shown by arrowheads).

The diabetes is a result of chronic pancreatitis. The most likely cause of the recurrent episodes of persistent hypoglycaemia is a poor glucagon response to low blood glucose levels, due to pancreatic destruction. Continuing alcohol abuse may be an alternative cause of frequent hypoglycaemia. Alcoholic liver disease may deplete glycogen stores and also reduce the response to hypoglycaemia.

Inflammation and irreversible fibrosis of the acini and ducts lead to pancreatic calcification and ductal lithiasis. The commonest cause above the age of 35 in the Western world is alcohol, followed by gallstones. Men are affected more than women. Other causes include hyperparathyroidism, hypertriglyceridaemia and ductal carcinoma. In the Far East, protein energy malnutrition is a major cause, and this has a younger age of onset and an equal sex distribution. Exocrine insufficiency leads to steatorrhoea, and should be treated with pancreatic supplements. Ductal carcinoma should be excluded, and complications such as pseudocyst or abscess formation may require surgery. This is also indicated for intractable pain. H_2-blockers and proton-pump inhibitors are also used to reduce pancreatic stimulation, together with vitamin supplements in cases of malabsorption.

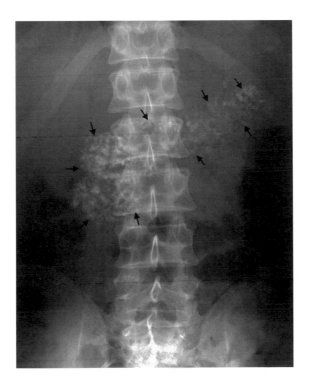

8

The ERCP shows (see below and opposite):
(a) intrahepatic duct dilation;
(b) a long stricture in the proximal common bile duct;
(c) a normal distal common bile duct;
(d) a normal pancreatic duct.

The likely diagnosis is cholangiocarcinoma. An alternative may be Caroli's disease.

In the Far East, cholangiocarcinoma appears to be associated with previous liver fluke infestation. There are two clinical forms: a peripheral form, in which nodules occur in both lobes of the liver; and a hilar form, which is situated at the confluence of right and left hepatic ducts. The tumour is locally invasive and occurs in the sixth or seventh decades of life, with men being affected more commonly than women. Survival is usually less than six months by the time a diagnosis is made. Hilar tumours are slow-growing, and can be stented to relieve obstruction or resected, with anastomotic reconstruction. Long-standing ulcerative colitis may also be associated with the above.

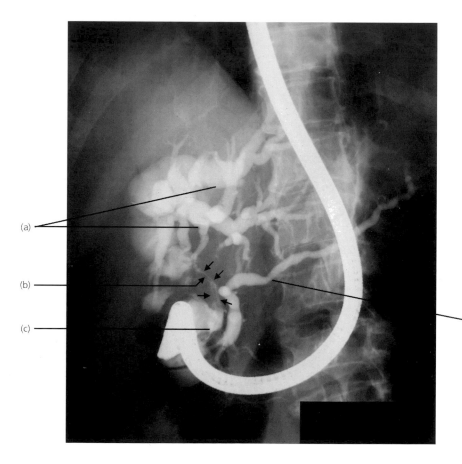

8

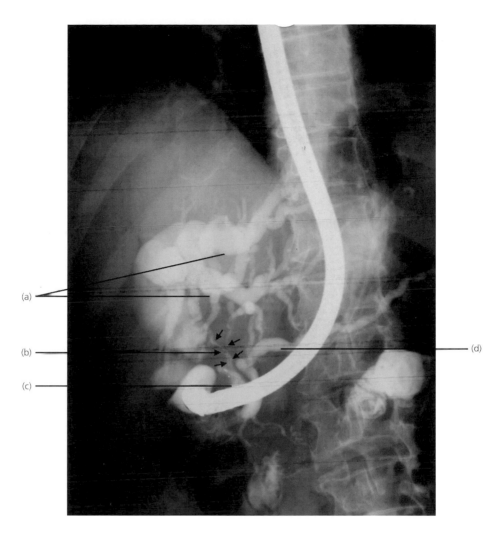

(a)

(b)

(c)

(d)

9

The ERCP shows (see overleaf):
(a) a dilated common bile duct;
(b) filling defects;
(c) dilated pancreatic duct.

The filling defects are multiple gallstones in the pancreatic duct, which are the cause of this woman's abdominal pain. Gallstones occur more commonly in women above the age of 40 who are obese and multiparous. Over 90% of stones are radiolucent. In this case, the obstruction can be resolved by sphincterotomy and stone removal using a Dormia basket. Large stones that cannot be removed may be suitable for lithotripsy.

9

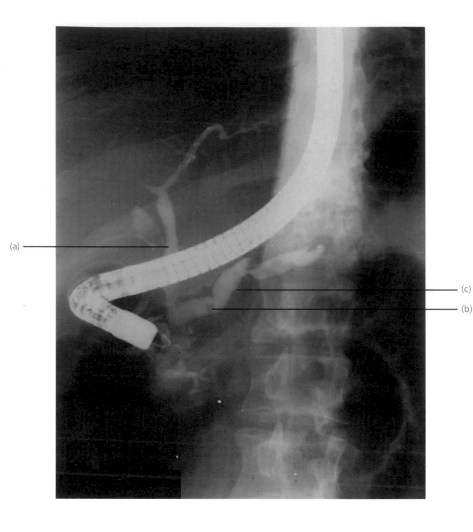

(a)

(c)

(b)

10

The CT scan of the abdomen shows (see opposite):
(a) a large mass in the right lobe of the liver (shown by arrowheads);
(b) cirrhosis of the liver;
(c) splenomegaly.

In view of the previous history of viral hepatitis and the history of unprotected intercourse, chronic hepatitis B carriage is probable. The absence of any other intra-abdominal pathology and the presence of a large mass in the liver makes the likely diagnosis primary hepatocellular cancer.

Hepatitis B is associated with an increased risk of hepatocellular cancer, especially in the Far East. The diagnosis may be confirmed by raised αFP (nearly all cases) and an ultrasound-guided or CT-guided biopsy. Cirrhosis is present in 80% of patients. Other aetiological factors are hepatitis C, any cause of cirrhosis, and aflatoxin derived from the

10 mould *Aspergillus flavus*. (The oral contraceptive pill has also been implicated.) Small tumours may be surgically resected (only 10% of cases); other techniques involve CT-guided phenol injections and cryotherapy. Chemotherapy with doxorubicin (20–30% respond), intra-arterial chemotherapy and embolization have also been tried, with varying success. The last option is orthotopic transplantation. The mean survival is four months.

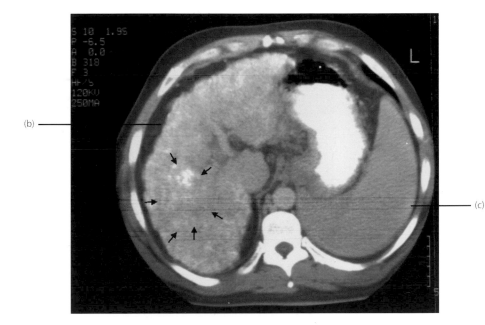

11 *The CT scan of the liver shows (see overleaf):*
(a) a large hypodense area within the liver;
(b) a fluid level within the mass;
(c) air in the bile ducts.

The diagnosis is a liver abscess. Liver abscesses occur secondary to biliary sepsis, portal pyaemia, generalized sepsis and occasionally intra-abdominal sepsis, e.g. a perforated duodenal ulcer or appendix. The organism is usually Gram-negative, and blood cultures are positive in 75% of cases.

A CXR in this situation would show:
(e) a raised right hemidiaphragm, with
(f) a reactive effusion.

11 Blood tests reveal a raised erythrocyte sedimentation rate (ESR) and white blood cell (WBC) count, and deranged U and Es (urea and electrolytes) and liver function tests (LFTs). Other diagnostic tests of use are ultrasound scanning or a ^{99m}Tc sulphur colloid uptake scan (rarely used). Treatment is with antibiotics and US-guided or CT-guided drainage.

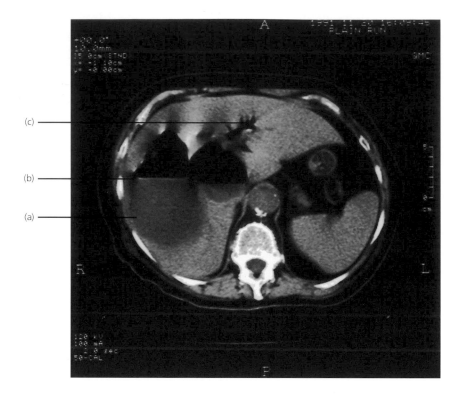

12 *The barium study shows (see opposite top):*
(a) gas-filled cysts in the walls of the large intestine. These may also be seen on a plain abdominal X-ray (*see opposite below*).

This is pneumatosis coli, which is associated with chronic obstructive pulmonary disease (COPD). The large gas-filled cysts contain mainly nitrogen. Occasionally, this condition is associated with peptic ulceration, or with pyloric obstruction. Usually, pneumatosis coli is asymptomatic, but occasionally it may cause pain, diarrhoea, tenesmus, obstruction and perforation. It is treated with hyperbaric O_2 therapy if required.

12

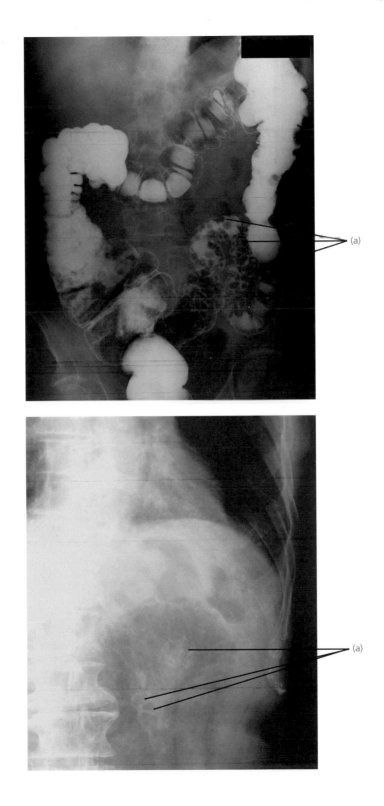

(a)

(a)

13

The barium study shows (see below and opposite top):
(a) a mass in the right side of the abdomen displacing the colon (shown by arrowheads).
(b) usually, multiple colonic polyps can be seen (not clear here).

The IVU shows (see opposite below):
(c) a mass on the right which is displacing the right kidney and causing obstruction.

The skull X-ray shows (see p. 232):
(d) osteomas of the mandible;

This is Gardner's syndrome, which consists of adenomatosis, a dermoid tumour of the abdomen, osteomas of the mandible and skull, sebaceous cysts and soft-tissue tumours of the skin. This is an autosomal dominant condition, a variant of congenital polyposis coli. Pressure or obstructive symptoms from large intra-abdominal dermoid tumours may require surgical relief. The colonic polyps should be managed as for familial adenomatous polyposis with regular screening, and panproctocolectomy should be considered before malignant transformation occurs. Severe bleeding from the polyps may also necessitate surgery.

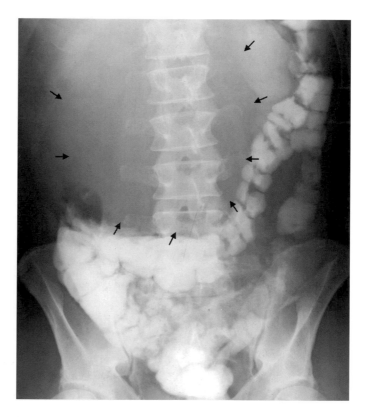

13

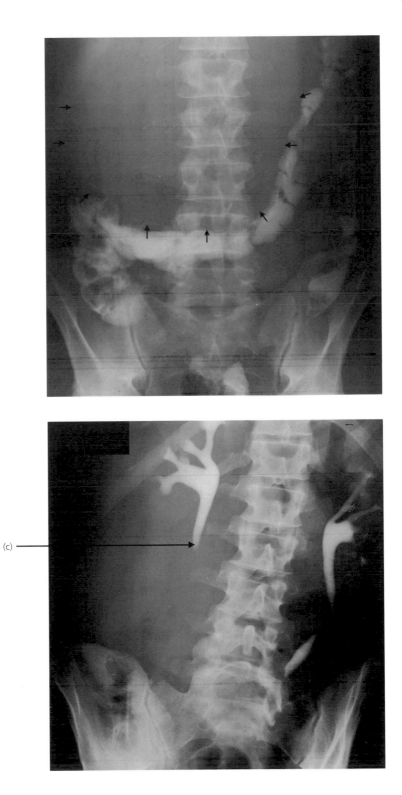

13

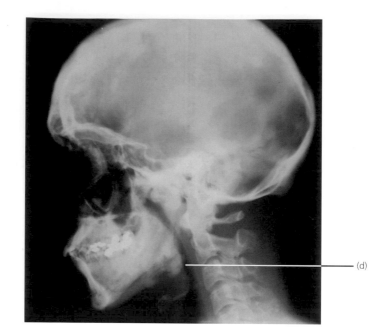

——— (d)

14

The barium swallow shows (see opposite):
(a) multiple large filling defects in the oesophagus;
(b) a serpiginous appearance due to submucosal filling defects (cf. the linear ulcers in Question 15). This is consistent with oesophageal varices.

This is a result of portal hypertension (portal pressure >12 mmHg). Portal hypertension can be divided into prehepatic, hepatic and post-hepatic forms. The majority of hepatic causes are due to cirrhosis (up to 50% have portal hypertension). Other hepatic causes are due to perisinusoidal diseases such as primary biliary cirrhosis (PBC), sarcoid and myeloproliferative disorders. Prehepatic causes include thrombosis or tumour invasion of the extrahepatic portal vein, leading to mechanical obstruction at this site. Post-hepatic causes are obstruction of the hepatic vein by thrombus (Budd–Chiari syndrome), or raised inferior vena caval pressure from right heart failure or constrictive pericarditis. Treatment of bleeding varices is by regular sclerotherapy or banding, and reducing portal pressure using propranolol or by inserting a porta-caval shunt.

14

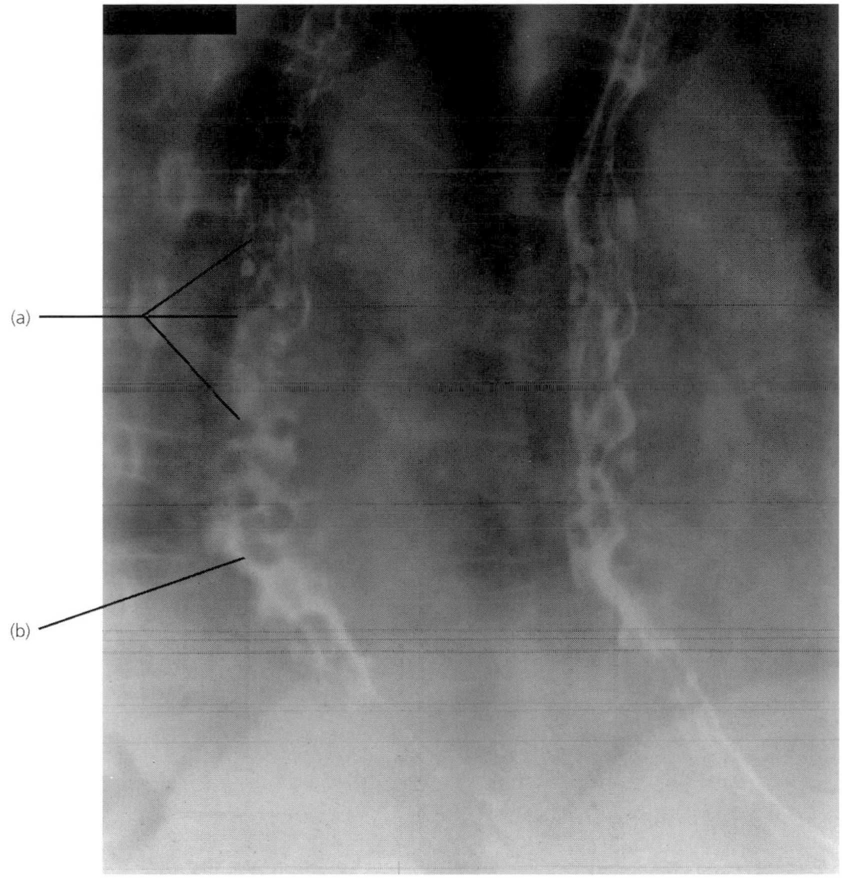

(a)

(b)

15

The barium swallow shows (see overleaf):
(a) a diffuse, net-like appearance affecting the majority of the oesophagus;
(b) punched-out ulcers, giving rise to a panoesophagitis.

The diagnosis is oesophageal candidiasis.

Herpes simplex and cytomegalovirus (CMV) infection may produce a similar appearance. The underlying cause here is acquired immuno-deficiency syndrome (AIDS), in view of the patient's previous history of drug abuse. Any cause of immunosuppression may give rise to oesophageal candidiasis. The commonest causes are chronic steroid usage, malignancy (especially leukaemia) either as a result of the disease itself or chemotherapy, alcohol abuse and diabetes.

15

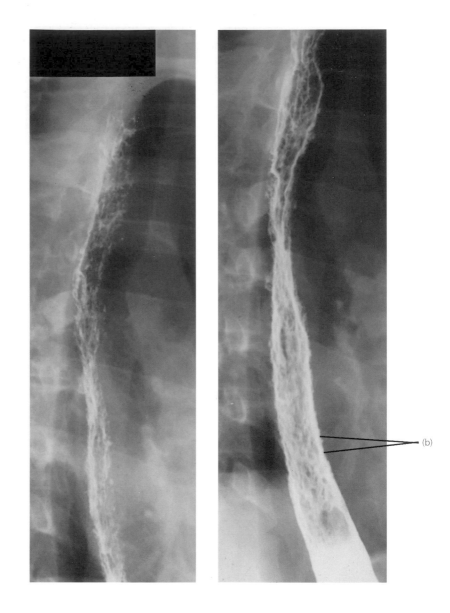

(b)

16

The barium swallow shows (see opposite and p. 236):
(a) a markedly dilated oesophagus with tapered narrowing at the gastro-oesophageal junction;
(b) food residue.

This is achalasia of the oesophagus, due to oesophageal dysmotility characterized by failure of the lower sphincter to relax and reduced oesophageal peristalsis. This leads to dilatation of the proximal portion

16

of the oesophagus and the retention of food. Patients complain of dysphagia, chest pain, regurgitation and weight loss. Aspiration of food contents leads to recurrent pneumonia. The differential diagnosis in the tropics is Chagas' disease, and in older patients cancer of the distal oesophagus. Treatment is by balloon dilation, botulinum toxin injection, or cardiomyotomy.

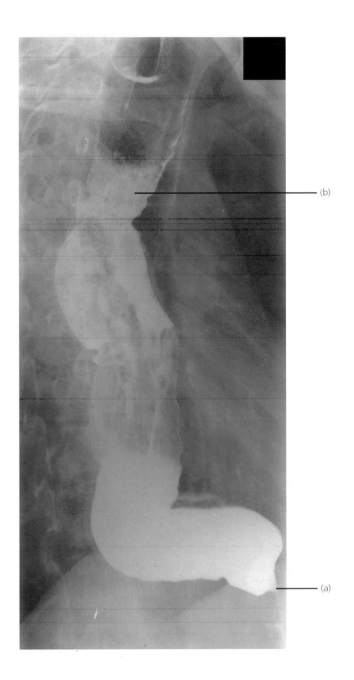

16

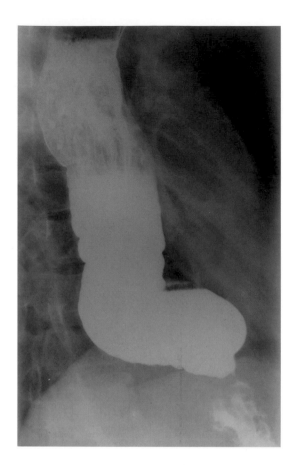

17

This is a double-contrast barium study, which shows (see opposite):
(a) a crater containing barium on the lesser curve.

This is the appearance of a gastric ulcer which, as it heals and fibroses, draws in the mucosal folds that can be seen.

Although this is likely to be benign, a gastroscopy should be carried out with biopsy or brush cytology to exclude malignancy. There is an association between gastric ulcers and *Helicobacter pylori* infection. *H. pylori* produces urease, which splits urea, and this is thought to stimulate gastrin and thus acid secretion. *H. pylori* can be detected by serology, the Clo test (which detects urease activity) and also the ^{14}C breath test. A number of eradication regimens are available. These involve the use of three or four agents, depending on the *H. pylori* sensitivity. These include antibiotics (amoxycillin, metronidazole, clarithromycin, tetracycline and tinidazole), proton-pump inhibitors and bismuth. The other major cause of benign gastric ulcers are non-

17 steroidal anti-inflammatory drugs (NSAIDs), which reduce prostacyclin production. Prostacyclin is thought to be cytoprotective and to affect local blood flow.

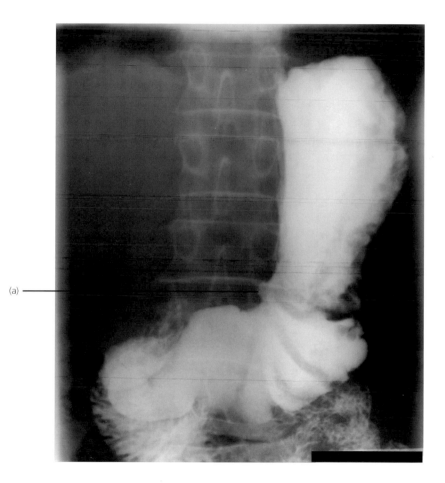

18 *The barium study shows (see overleaf and p. 239 top):*
(a) a duodenal ulcer crater;
(b) distorted mucosa with radiating folds in the duodenal caps, suggesting that the condition is chronic (shown by arrowheads).

The plain X-ray shows (see p. 239 bottom):
(c) pneumoperitoneum, probably due to a perforated duodenal ulcer.

This patient has had a perforated ulcer despite H_2-receptor blockade and this raises the possibility of the Zollinger–Ellison (ZE) syndrome. A raised fasting gastrin level will help confirm the diagnosis.

18

The unifying diagnosis in this woman is MEN type 1 (Werner's syndrome). This is an autosomal dominant condition characterized by tumours of the anterior pituitary, parathyroid and pancreatic islets. The presence of a raised calcium level and a prolactinoma would support this diagnosis.

Gastrinomas can be imaged by a highly selective digital subtraction angiography (DSA) scan, and most occur in the body or tail of the pancreas. Around 95% are associated with peptic ulceration and 40% with diarrhoea. The administration of secretin reduces gastrin secretion in normal people, but in the ZE syndrome gastrin levels are paradoxically increased, and this provides the basis for the secretin test. ZE syndrome is treated with high-dose proton-pump inhibition, and surgery is used in cases of medical failure. In malignant cases, the patients are treated with streptozotocin.

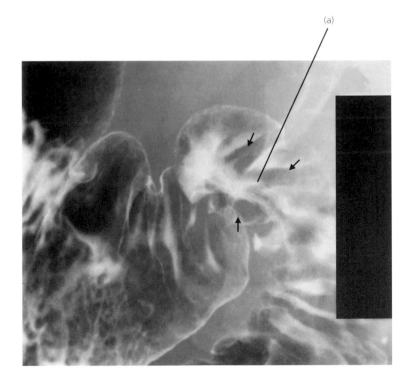

(a)

18

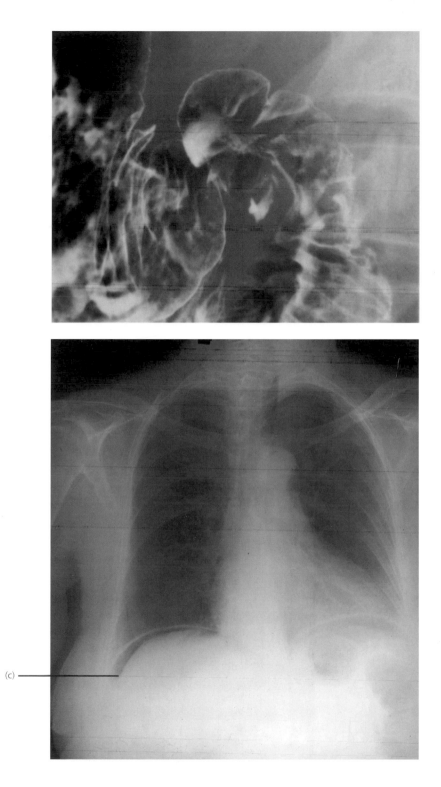

(c)

19

The barium follow-through shows:
(a) multiple mucosal outpouching from the mesenteric border of the jejunum (shown by arrowheads).

These are jejunal diverticula. The cause of her anaemia is vitamin B_{12} or folate deficiency.

The muscle weakness is caused by hypocalcaemia.

Bacterial overgrowth, which is common in jejunal diverticula, has led to malabsorption of vitamin D and calcium, and therefore to muscle weakness. The bacteria also break down folate and vitamin B_{12}, and this leads to a macrocytic anaemia. Bacterial overgrowth can be confirmed by the hydrogen breath test after giving lactulose or glucose. Small-bowel diverticula develop secondary to intestinal dysmotility and connective-tissue disease, e.g. systemic sclerosis and Marfan's syndrome. Patients are usually asymptomatic, but on bacterial colonization they develop malabsorption, which can be confirmed by measuring faecal fats and using the xylose test (carbohydrate malabsorption). Treatment is empirical, with tetracycline or metronidazole. If this fails, jejunal aspiration is recommended to identify the organism.

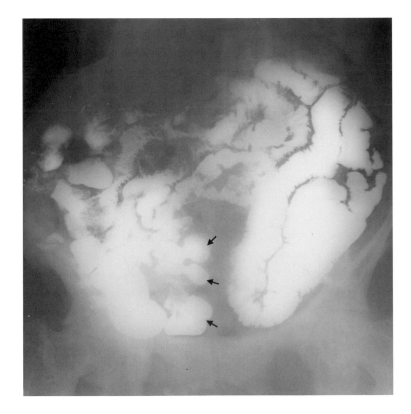

20

The barium study shows:
(a) a long filling defect in an otherwise normal intestine.

This is *Ascaris lumbricoides* (roundworm) infestation (ascariasis). This is a common condition in Asia, Africa and Central America, and affects mainly children. Ingestion of eggs, which subsequently grow in the body, leads to a variety of symptoms, such as fever, urticaria, malaise and abdominal colic.

Migration of larvae through the lungs leads to pneumonitis and marked bronchospasm. A CXR should be done if patients describe SOB or wheezing. It would show:
(b) marked mottling across the lung fields;
(c) peribronchial marking.

This is known as Löffler's syndrome. A full blood count should be done, which will show marked eosinophilia.

Occasionally, a large bolus of worms in the intestines leads to intestinal obstruction. They may also infest the common bile duct and the liver, causing cholangitis, biliary obstruction and hepatic infestation. Treatment is with mebendazole, levamisole and piperazine salts. Surgery is indicated for obstruction.

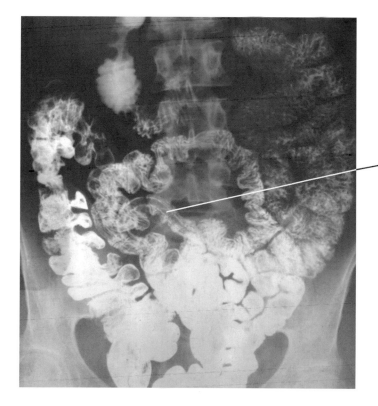

(a)

21

The plain abdominal X-ray shows:
(a) intramural gas throughout the small intestine. This represents necrotic bowel (shown by arrowheads).

The diagnosis is acute ischaemia of the small intestine. Perforation, haemorrhage and secondary infection are common. Surgery with resection of ischaemic bowel offers the only chance of survival. In chronic cases, vascular insufficiency leads to stricture formation. The commonest sites are watershed areas like the splenic flexure. There is an increased incidence of mesenteric ischaemia in people with AF or evidence of atherosclerosis affecting other organs. Prognosis from acute ischaemia is poor, with less than 20% survival rate.

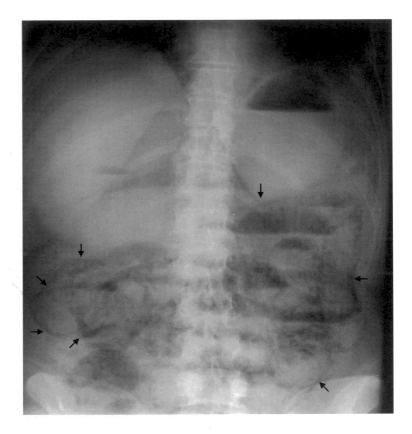

22

The barium study shows (see opposite):
(a) a narrowed, rigid stomach with an intact mucosa.

This is known as 'leather bottle stomach', or linitis plastica. This is a gastric carcinoma with widespread submucosal invasion that gives rise

22

to this rigid appearance. The condition occurs in younger patients, and the prognosis is poor. Tumours associated with intestinal metaplasia occur in older patients, and are often polypoid. The most frequent site is the antrum of the stomach. The prognosis is slightly better in this group.

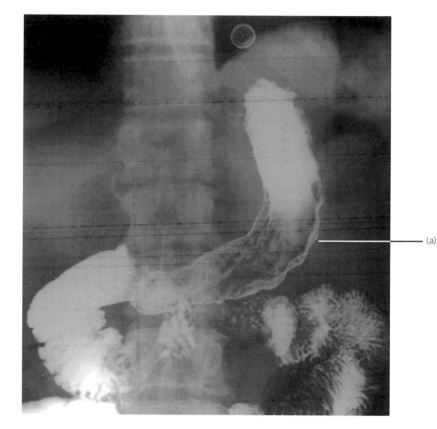

— (a)

23

The barium enema shows (see overleaf top and bottom):
(a) an apple-core stenosis in the ascending colon;
(b) the passage of barium and air into the duodenum.

This represents colonic carcinoma with fistula formation. Weight loss and anaemia would be the initial presentation of right-sided colonic tumours, but subsequent fistula formation leads to the passage of faeculent products into the duodenum and stomach, giving rise to the symptoms described. Left-sided colonic tumours give rise to obstructive symptoms.

23

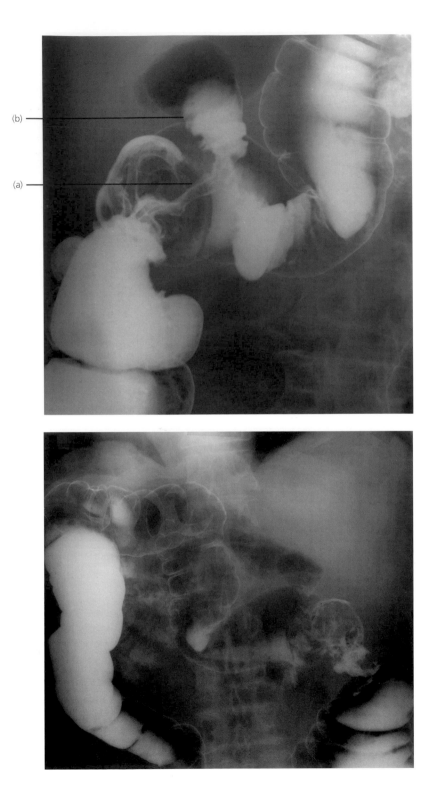

24

The plain X-ray shows:
(a) gas under the right hemidiaphragm.

In the given clinical context, this appearance represents a subphrenic abscess. These arise secondary to intra-abdominal sepsis, often from a perforation, e.g. of the appendix or gallbladder. Malaise, fever and shoulder-tip pain may be the only findings. The radiological appearance above is often accompanied by a reactive pericardial effusion, and screening of the diaphragm shows impaired movement. Treatment is by antibiotics and surgical drainage.

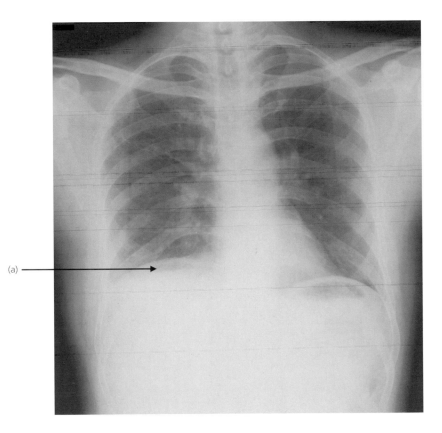

(a)

Haematology

The chest X-ray shows (see below):
(a) enlargement of the mediastinal lymph nodes;
(b) right lower lobe pneumonia.

The diagnosis is Hodgkin's lymphoma.
   Useful tests include a CT scan of the chest and abdomen and a bone marrow trephine, for accurate staging of the lymphoma. A tissue biopsy is required for grading.

The CT scan of the abdomen shows (see opposite):
(c) para-aortic lymphadenopathy.

It may also show (not in this example):
(d) echogenic areas in the liver;
(e) echogenic areas in the spleen.

This is the most common type of lymphoma, and it has a bimodal age distribution, with the first peak occurring in early adult life and a second

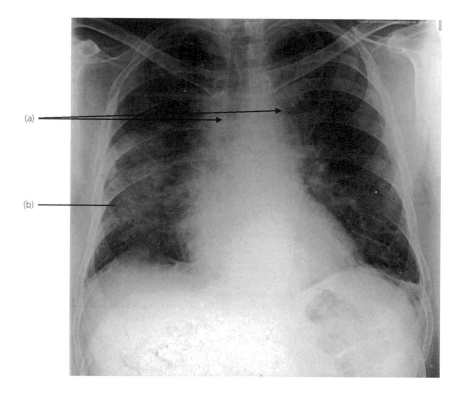

1

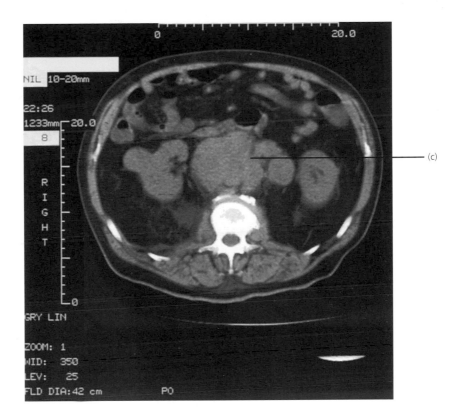

in those in their mid-40s. Patients are staged using the revised Ann Arbor classification, which is based on the lymph-node areas involved and whether the patients have symptoms such as weight loss, fever and sweating (stage B). Treatment varies from radiotherapy for stage Ia and stage IIa patients, to chemotherapy for Stage Ib and IIb onwards. Supportive treatment is also important.

2

The X-ray shows (see overleaf):
(a) frontal bossing of the skull;
(b) expansion of the maxilla;
   The X-ray could also show:
(c) the so-called 'hair-on-end appearance'.

The diagnosis is β-thalassaemia major. This boy will have been inadequately transfused during early life. Diagnosis is difficult once the boy is on a transfusion regimen, but it is possible by gene analysis of a pre-transfusion blood sample, or by examination of the parents' blood.

   This is an anaemia caused by an absence or impairment in the production of beta chains. The alpha chains combine with any available gamma

2

and delta chains to form haemoglobin F and haemoglobin A$_2$, respectively. The thalassaemias can be divided clinically into thalassaemia major, thalassaemia intermedia and thalassaemia minor, and they correlate with the severity of the anaemia. Extramedullary haematopoiesis is a typical feature of the patient who is inadequately transfused, leading to expansion of bone marrow and hepatosplenomegaly.

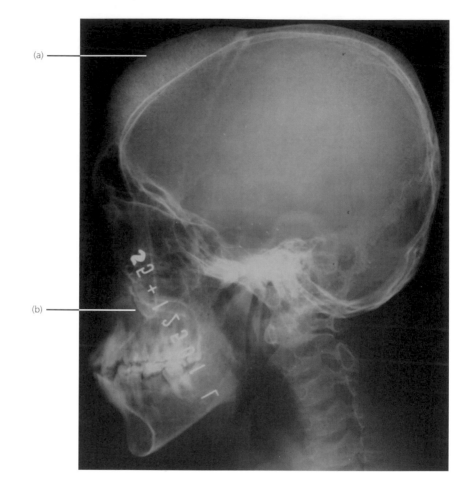

(a)

(b)

3

The X-rays show (see opposite, p. 250 & p. 251):
(a) expansion of the marrow;
(b) thinning of the cortex;
(c) the bones appear osteoporotic.

This is a typical appearance of β-thalassaemia in a patient previously inadequately transfused. Chronic haemolysis and recurrent transfusions

3

lead to iron overload. Deposition of excess iron in the endocrine glands leads to impaired secretion of various hormones, e.g. insulin, which in this case led to diabetes. This could have been prevented by the use of desferrioxamine as a chelating agent. If the spleen is enlarged, its removal can reduce transfusion requirements and reduce iron overload.

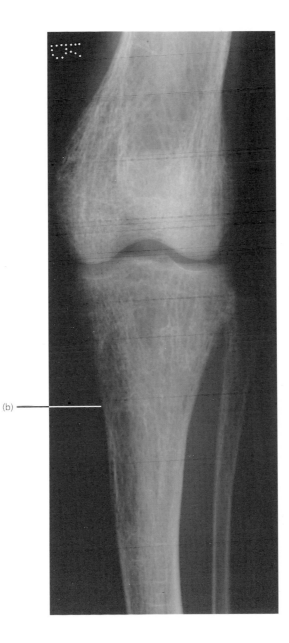

(b)

3

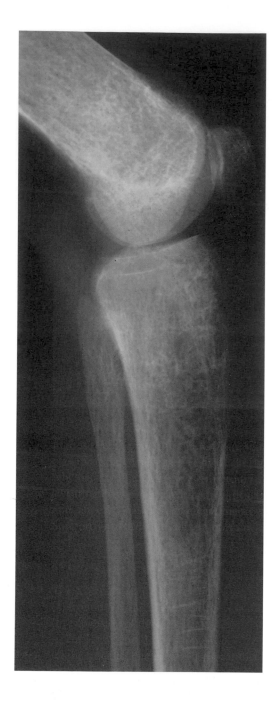

3

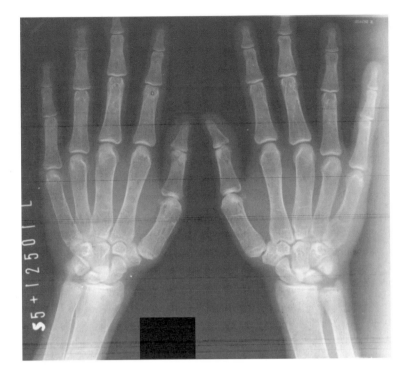

4

The lateral skull X-ray shows (see overleaf):
(a) multiple lytic lesions (shown by arrowheads).

Such lesions on the skull lead to the so-called 'pepper-pot skull' appearance. The diagnosis is multiple myeloma.

The diagnosis can be confirmed by the presence of paraproteinaemia on serum immunoelectrophoresis and/or the presence of Bence-Jones protein in the urine; by bone marrow aspiration showing an increase in plasma cell infiltrate; or, finally, by a skeletal survey (not bone scan) looking for multiple lytic lesions at different sites. Two out of three of these tests are required to make a diagnosis, and the presence of lytic lesions or a paraprotein level >30 g/L makes the diagnosis likely.

Patients may present with infections due to immunosuppression, or back pain due to vertebral collapse, leading to loss of height and possible paraplegia. Renal failure due to light-chain deposition or hypercalcaemia is also a not uncommon presentation. Prognostic markers are bone lesions, level of monoclonal protein, anaemia, hypercalcaemia, albumin, β_2-microglobulin, IL-6 level and age.

4

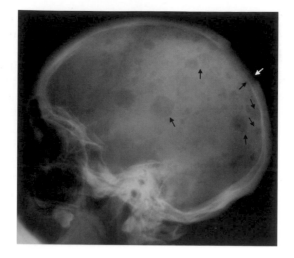

5

The X-ray shows:
(a) narrowing of the joint space;
(b) irregular erosions;
(c) cyst formation and sclerosis;
(d) overgrowth of the epiphysis;
(e) widened squared intercondylar notches.
  The X-ray could also show:
(f) synovial thickening (not shown here).

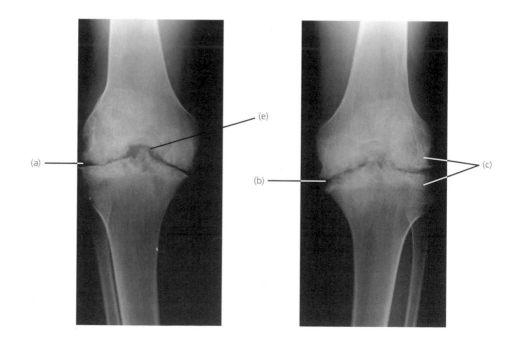

5

The diagnosis is haemophilia A with recurrent haemarthrosis of the knee joint. This in turn leads to a chronic arthropathy. (Haemophilia B would present similarly.)

Haemophilia A is inherited as an X-linked trait, and is characterized by a depletion in factor VIIIC. The bleeding time and prothrombin time are normal, but the activated thromboplastin time is increased. Bleeding is treated by intravenous administration of factor VIII as a concentrate. In order to treat haemarthrosis, levels of factor VIII above 30% are aimed for. Other procedures, such as surgery or dental extraction, require levels above 50%. Desmopressin (DDAVP) can increase low levels of factor VIII and can be used to treat bleeds in mild to moderate haemophilia. There was formerly a danger of acquiring hepatitis B or C from blood products, as in this case, but this has been all but eliminated by present surveillance methods.

6

This MRI coronal T1-weighted image shows (see below and overleaf):
(a) bilateral areas of subcortical infarction in the femoral heads;
(b) a clear zone of demarcation, which implies this is in the healing phase.

This is typical of avascular necrosis of the femoral head. In this age group, recurrent episodes of sickling in the vasculature of the femoral head lead to this appearance. An alternative diagnosis would be previous treatment with high-dose steroids, such as is used in the treatment of

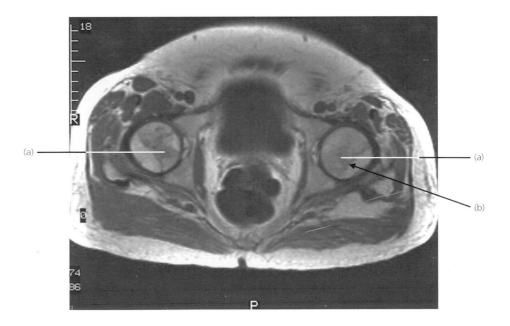

6

high-grade non-Hodgkin's lymphoma and acute lymphoblastic lymphoma. The cause in this Afro-Caribbean patient is sickle-cell disease due to homozygous Hb SS, Hb SC disease, or Hb S β-thalassaemia.

Sickle-cell disease is confirmed by Hb electrophoresis. Sickle cells can be seen on a peripheral blood film, and the presence of Hb S can be readily confirmed by the sodium metabisulphite test. Patients with sickle-cell disease have a chronic haemolytic state. Sickling crises are precipitated by infections, dehydration and hypoxia. This leads to vaso-occlusion and infarction of spleen, bone, retina, and kidney. These patients are more susceptible to infections with *Salmonella* and encapsulated organisms such as pneumococci. It is therefore current practice to vaccinate these patients with Pneumovax.

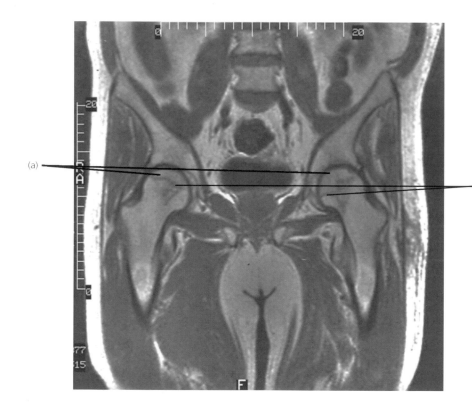

Neurology

1

This is an MRI scan of the neck, which shows (see below):
(a) a central syrinx in the cervical cord;
(b) herniation of the cerebellar tonsils through the foramen magnum.

The diagnosis is syringomyelia, with an Arnold–Chiari malformation. For comparison, the next scan (*see overleaf*) shows collapse of the syrinx after surgery (c).

A fluid-filled cavity (syrinx) in the central cord produces signs of a lower motor neurone (LMN) lesion at the level of the lesion, with wasting of the muscles of the hand, and loss of reflexes. There are signs of an upper motor neurone (UMN) lesion in the legs, with brisk reflexes and extensor plantars. Loss of pain and temperature occurs in a band across the chest, at the level of the syrinx. As the lesion expands, sensory loss extends to cover the chest, arms and finally the head in a 'balaclava' distribution (syringobulbia). Sensory loss in the upper limbs leads to the development of neuropathic joints in the shoulders and elbows. Spastic paraparesis may occur at this stage. Syringomyelia may be associated with a number of skeletal abnormalities.

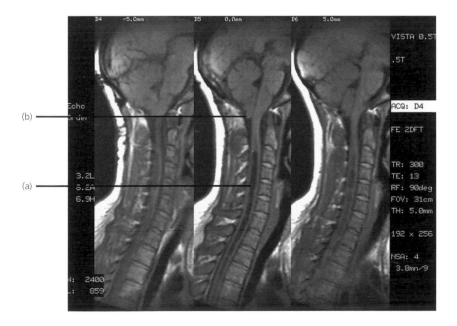

1

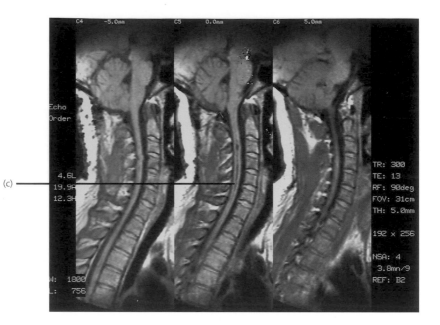

2

The CT scan shows (see opposite top):

(a) a hypodense area (subdural haematoma), which is probably three or four weeks old;

(b) midline shift to the left;

(c) compression of the lateral ventricles;

(d) obliteration of the sulci on the right in comparison with the left.

Due to red cell and protein breakdown, the fluid in the subdural space appears hypodense. This appearance should be compared with that of an acute subdural-haematoma (*see opposite bottom*). In this image, no contrast has been added, but a high attenuation area appears in the subdural space (e). Note that the medial border is concave, compared with an acute extradural haematoma (f), where it is convex (*see p. 258*). Acute extradural haematomas occur more commonly in a younger age group, usually as a result of damage to the meningeal arteries. In the last example, active bleeding, mixed with areas of clot, gives rise to mixed attenuation signals on the CT. These cases require urgent neurosurgical intervention.

Subdural haematomas are caused by deceleration head injuries, e.g. falls, and are more common in people with cerebral atrophy. This results in a tearing of the veins that bridge the cortex and the sagittal sinus. Presenting symptoms include drowsiness, headaches, mild intellectual impairment and a fluctuating conscious level. In patients with cerebral atrophy, e.g. the elderly or alcoholics, the presentation may be several months after the precipitating event. About 20% of cases are bilateral.

2   Extradural haematomas arise from a tear of the middle meningeal artery or one of its branches, usually secondary to a skull fracture. Patients describe a transient loss of consciousness, followed by a lucid interval. Progressive hemiparesis and stupor follow. Initially, there is

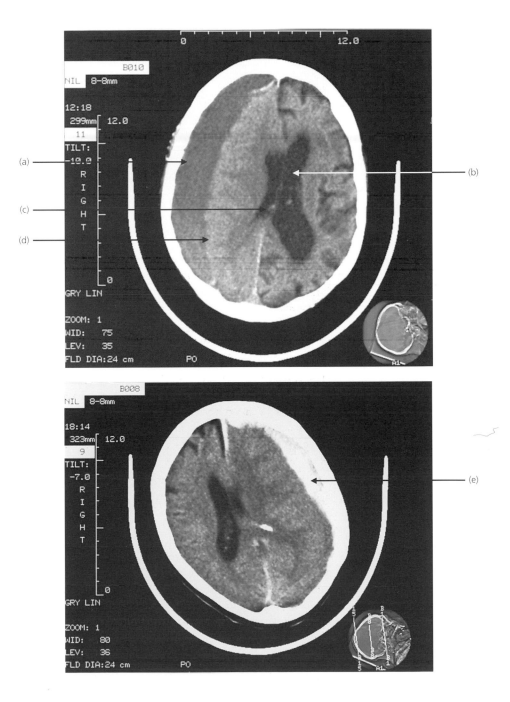

2

an ipsilateral dilated pupil followed by bilateral fixed dilated pupils and tetraplegia. The signs are due to the rapid accumulation of blood in a closed cavity. Acute subdural haematomas present in a similar manner.

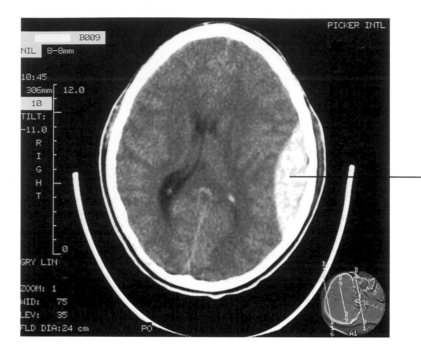

3

This is a CT study of the head which shows (see opposite):
(a) a mass in the frontal lobe with an area of low density around it (oedema).
(b) After contrast administration, an area of ring enhancement around the mass can be seen. This represents a hyperaemic area around the mass.
(c) The mass is smooth and thin-walled.

The diagnosis is a cerebral abscess, which classically presents adjacent to the frontal sinus and may often be multiple. A differential diagnosis would be cerebral metastases.

This is caused by a localized collection of pus, which may have been the result of a penetrating head injury, spread of local infection, e.g. mastoiditis, sinusitis, and haematogenous spread. Treatment involves surgical drainage; steroids to reduce surrounding oedema; and intravenous antibiotics.

3

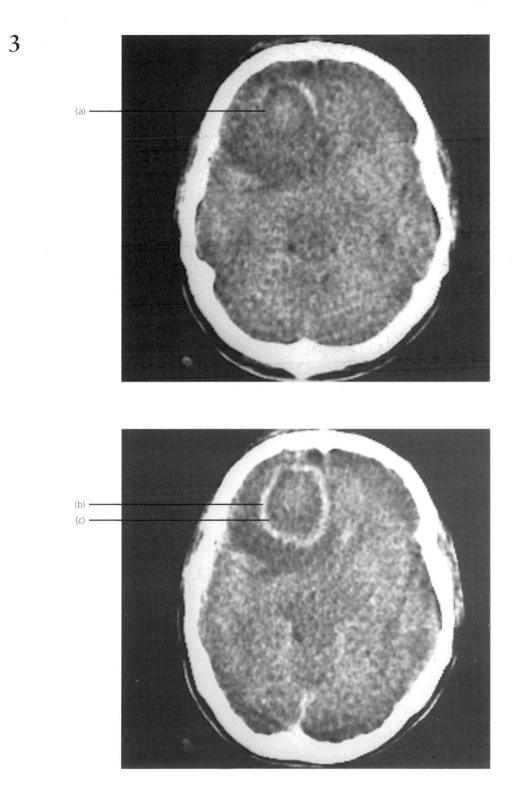

(a)

(b)
(c)

4   *This is a carotid arteriogram, which shows:*
(a) an enlarged feeding vessel;
(b) a tangle of abnormal vessels of variable sizes;
(c) an early venous blush during the arterial phase;
(d) an abnormally enlarged vein.

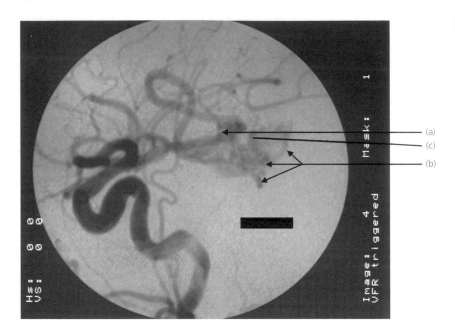

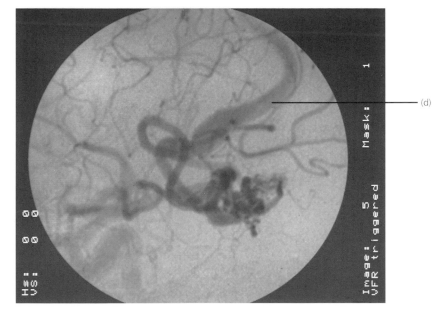

4

This is a large AV malformation. These present in several ways: firstly, haemorrhage, which may be subarachnoid or intracerebral. This tends to be less severe, and there is a smaller rebleeding rate compared to bleeds from aneurysms. Intracerebral bleeds tend to present with focal symptoms and signs. Secondly, patients may present with a fit during a bleed, or increasing frequency of seizures due to an increase in the size of the AV malformation, or rarely due to an intracerebral 'steal phenomenon'. Patients may also be conscious of turbulent blood flow and describe 'rushing noises' in their heads. Treatment involves embolization, or stereotactic radiotherapy.

5

The CT scan shows (see below & overleaf top):
(a) blood in the basal cisterns and the Sylvian fissure.

The angiogram shows (see overleaf bottom):
(b) an aneurysm of the posterior communicating artery (shown by arrows).

The patient has presented with a subarachnoid haemorrhage. CT does not always confirm the diagnosis, and a lumbar puncture looking for xanthochromia by spectrophotometry may be required. Typically, an angiogram identifies the site of the aneurysm. Intracranial aneurysms may occur at a number of sites, and the example below (*see p. 263 top*) shows an anterior communicating artery aneurysm (c).

Treatment is by surgically clipping the aneurysm or endovascular embolization (*see p. 263 bottom*), e.g., for a vertebral artery aneurysm (d).

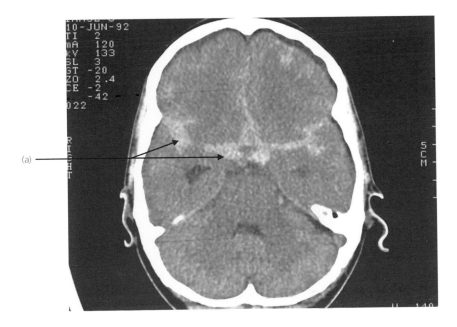

5   There is a high rate of rebleeding without intervention. Around 5% of patients rebleed within 24 hours, another 20% within two weeks and

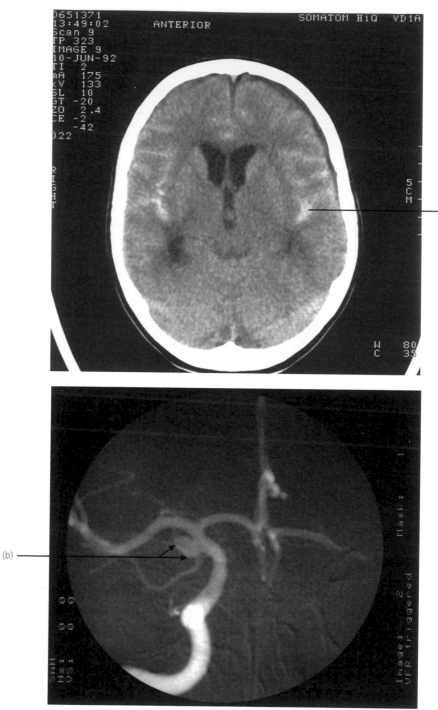

5

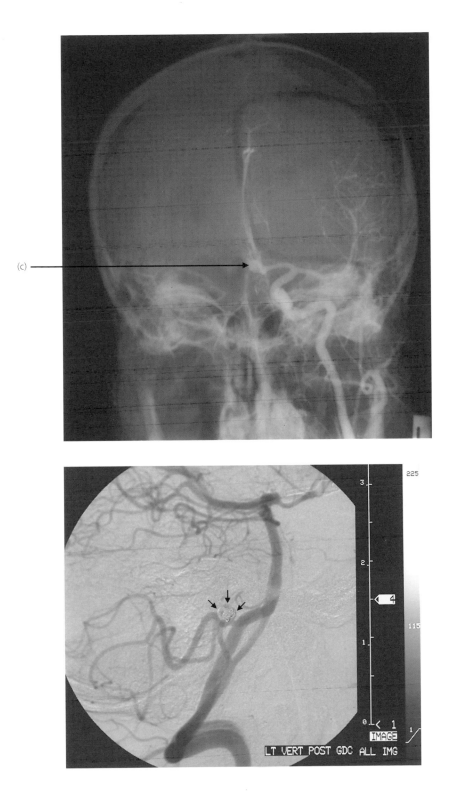

(c)

LT VERT POST GDC ALL IMG

5 50% by six months. Calcium antagonists such as nimodipine are also used to reduce cerebral vascular spasm and hence ischaemia.

6 *The skull X-ray shows*:
(a) serpiginous lines (shown by arrowheads).

These are caused by calcification of brain parenchyma. The calcifications underlie angiomas of the pia mater. The diagnosis is Sturge–Weber syndrome. Other features are capillary haemangiomas in the distribution of the ophthalmic division of the trigeminal nerve, mental retardation, epilepsy, hemiparesis and rarely glaucoma. A CT scan would show:
(b) cerebral atrophy;
(c) calcification of cerebral angiomas;
(d) calcification of the cerebral cortex, especially in the occipitoparietal region.

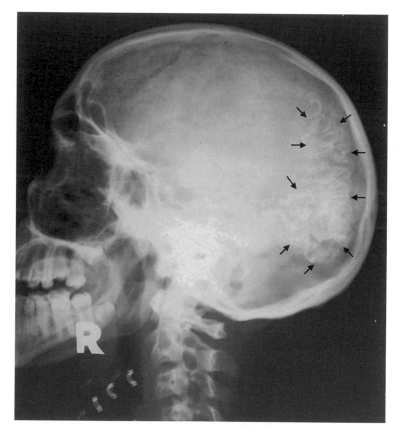

7 *The CT scan, with contrast, shows* (*see opposite*):
(a) well-circumscribed ovoid areas, which are densely enhancing and well demarcated (shown by arrowheads);
(b) they lie adjacent to the dura mater;

7

(c) they occupy the parafalcine area;
(d) and also the sphenoid ridge.

These are meningiomas. An alternative differential diagnosis would be cerebral metastases. Meningiomas are slow-growing benign tumours arising from the arachnoid mater. They are well vascularized, and are supplied by the external carotid artery. Note the rich vascular supply of the meningioma (vascular blush) (e) (*see arrowheads overleaf top*). They can occasionally erode bone, and may be seen as calcified lesions on a skull X-ray (hyperostosis) (f) (*see arrowheads overleaf bottom and p. 267*).

Patients may present with partial seizures, focal neurological signs, or with symptoms of raised intracranial pressure.

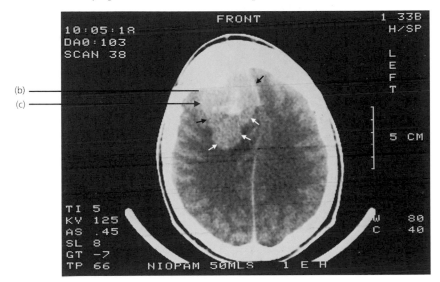

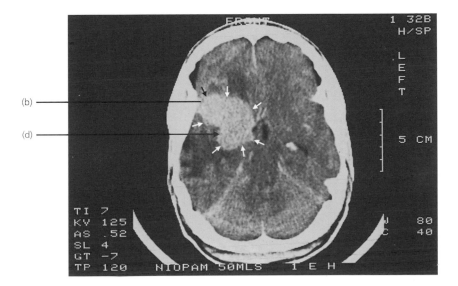

7

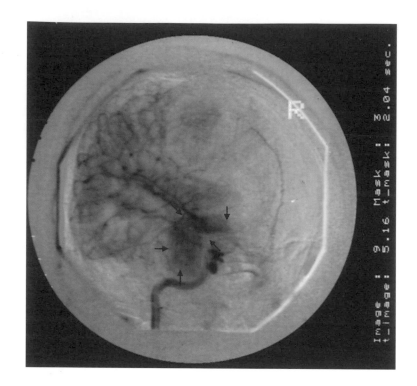

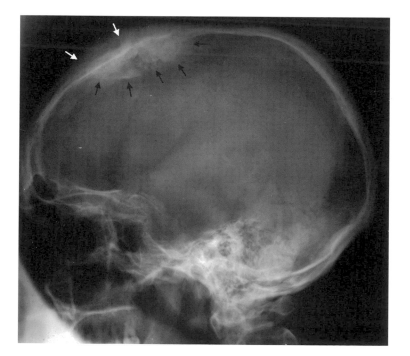

7

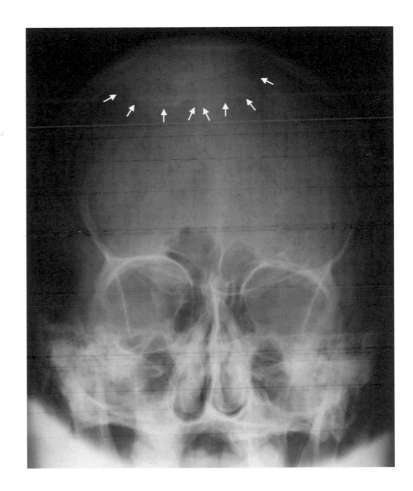

8

The MRI scan shows (*see overleaf top*):
(a) bilateral masses in the region of the cerebellopontine angle (shown by arrowheads).

This is a bilateral acoustic neuroma. A differential diagnosis would be a meningioma. Involvement of cranial nerve:
VIII—results in progressive deafness, tinnitus, vestibular disturbance;
VII—results in facial weakness (rare);
V—results in loss of facial sensation (especially the corneal reflex).
Ipsilateral cerebellar signs also occur, and if the tumour exerts pressure on the brainstem, ipsilateral UMN signs such as hyperreflexia may be seen.

A smaller unilateral acoustic neuroma (b) (*see overleaf bottom*) would present with sensorineural deafness.

Seventy per cent of tumours arise from Schwann cells. When neuromas occurs bilaterally, it is usually a neurofibroma, and there is associated neurofibromatosis. Brainstem evoked potentials pick up

8

abnormalities in over 90% of cases of acoustic neuroma. Early surgery may preserve cranial nerve function, but large tumours are associated with a high morbidity.

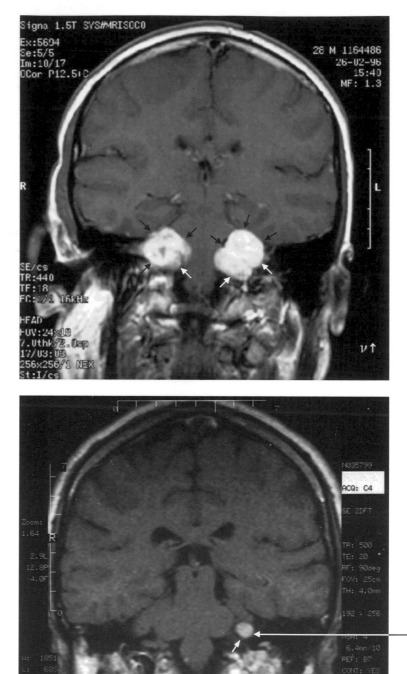

(b)

9

The MRI scan shows (see below):
(a) elongated enhancing area within the cervical cord;
(b) no expansion of the cord around this area.

The MRI scan of the head of the same patient taken 18 months later shows (see overleaf):
(c) multiple periventricular white matter plaques. These represent areas of demyelination, which can be further enhanced with gadolinium, and give an appearance of 'Roman candles' (shown by arrowheads).

The diagnosis is multiple sclerosis. In this example, the patient may have presented with acute cord dysfunction at C4–C5. Differential diagnoses of the cervical spine image include transverse myelitis, meningeal disease and tumours. Multiple sclerosis is a demyelinating disorder of unknown aetiology. Patients present with neurological symptoms and signs at different levels, separated in time and space. Common presentations are difficulty in walking, spastic paraparesis, bladder symptoms and cerebellar ataxia. Oligoclonal immunoglobulin bands in the cerebrospinal fluid (CSF) and MRI scans of the head are used to confirm the diagnosis. Treatment is supportive, with short courses of methylprednisolone for acute relapses. Early trials of interferon-β also show promise.

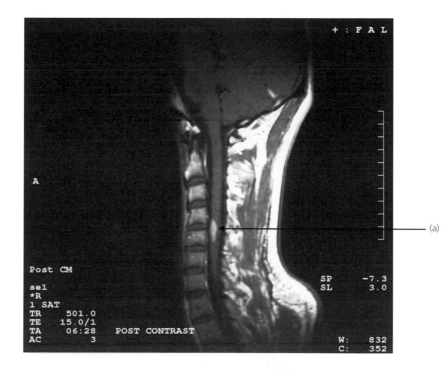

9

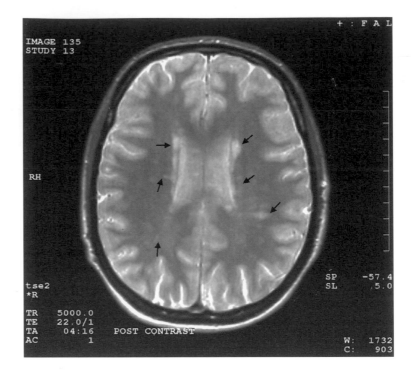

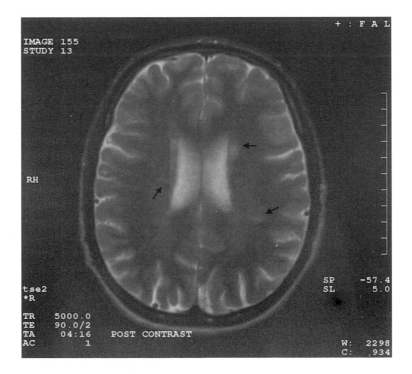

10

The CT scan shows (see below top):
(a) calcification of hamartomatous lesions in the periventricular area;
(b) a giant-cell astrocytoma (benign) at the end of the third ventricle, near the foramen of Monro.

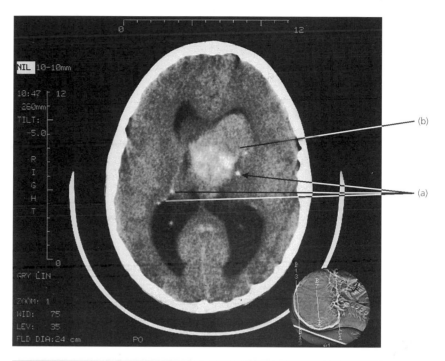

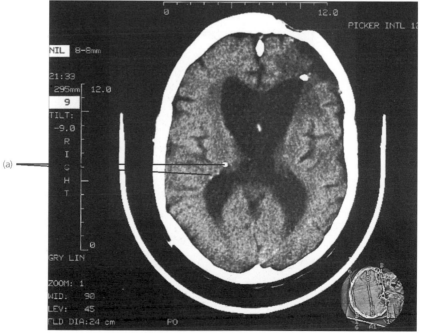

10

The CT scan (*see p. 271 bottom*) shows the same patient after surgery. The hamartomatous lesions remain, but the giant-cell astrocytoma has now been removed.

The diagnosis is tuberous sclerosis or epiloia. This is an autosomal dominant condition characterized by mental retardation and epilepsy.

There are a number of cutaneous features, which include adenoma sebaceum over the face, ash-leaf patches (white oval areas of depigmentation) over the thorax, and raised naevi, which have an oily appearance around the spine (shagreen patches). Management involves treatment of epilepsy and genetic counselling.

The initial neurological signs are commonly found in postictal patients, and are not a manifestation of the underlying disease.

11

This is an axial uncontrasted CT scan which shows (see below, p. 273 and p. 274 top):
(a) high attenuation near the superior sagittal sinus, representing thrombus;
(b) subcortical haemorrhage in the left parietal grey matter. This is typical of haemorrhagic venous infarction.

This is a late-phase cerebral angiogram which shows (see p. 274 bottom):
(c) a filling defect in the posterior aspect of the superior sagittal sinus, with;
(d) contrast around it.

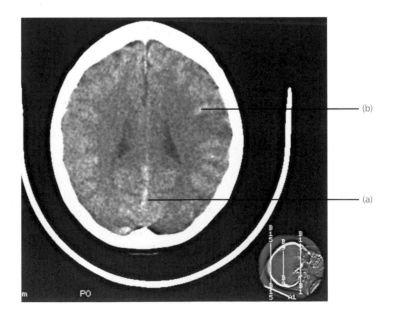

11

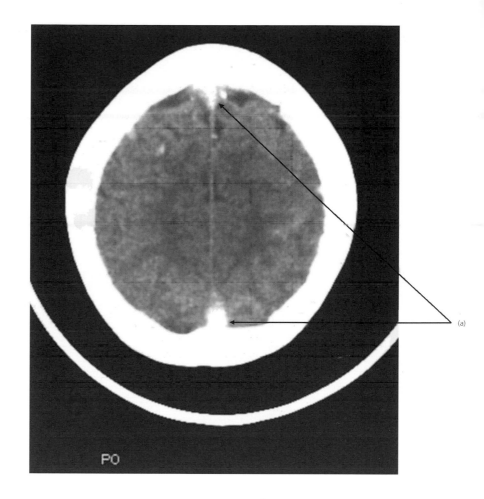

(a)

In this case, dehydration has led to venous thrombosis. The classical delta sign is seen in only around 30% of cases. This leads to symptoms of raised intracranial pressure, and occasionally fits. Infection involving the face, e.g. orbital cellulitis, may lead to an ascending thrombophlebitis and hence thrombosis of the venous sinuses that are involved. Thus, orbital infection leads to cavernous sinus thrombosis, leading to ocular pain, proptosis and chemosis. Papilloedema and an ophthalmoplegia often occur. Middle ear infections tend to lead to lateral sinus thrombosis. Cortical venous thrombosis leads to focal signs and even hemiplegia. Venous thrombosis is associated with coagulation disorders, pregnancy and the use of the contraceptive pill. The diagnosis is confirmed by either CT, MRI or DSA scans.

Treatment involves intravenous antibiotics, anticoagulant therapy and rehydration.

11

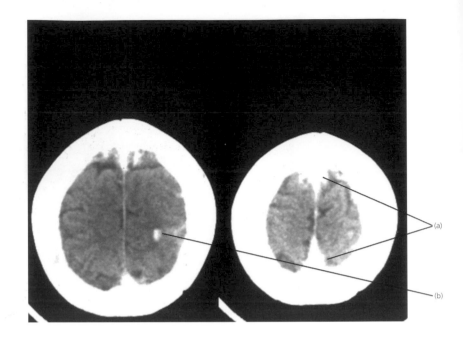

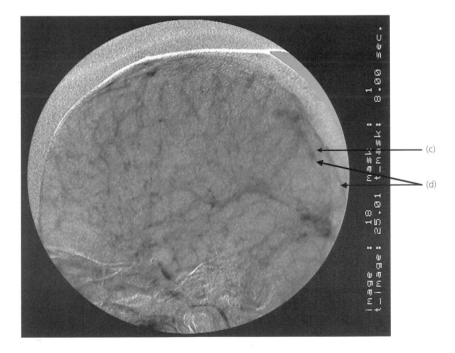

12

The CT scan shows:

(a) an irregular hyperdense, post-contrast lesion in the right basal ganglia (*shown by arrowheads, see below*);

(b) a similar lesion in the left occipital area (*shown by arrowheads, see overleaf*).

This is cerebral toxoplasmosis, complicating AIDS. These lesions are not thin-walled, and do not enhance well. A differential diagnosis is cerebritis. When healed, they appear as multiple calcified areas. The differential diagnosis in such cases is TB.

Typically, patients present with confusion, lethargy, altered conscious level and seizures. Focal signs may be present. Treatment is with pyrimethamine and sulphadiazine. Specific IgM or a four-fold rise in antibody titre over 4 weeks implies acute infection. Lymph node or brain biopsy may be diagnostic.

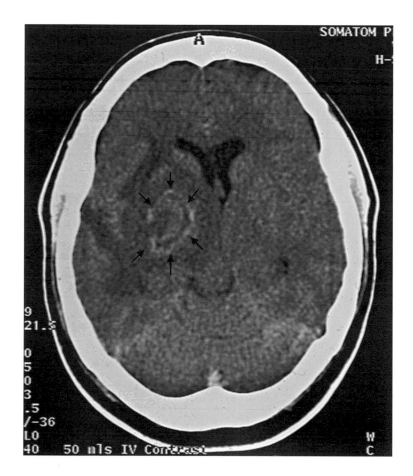

12

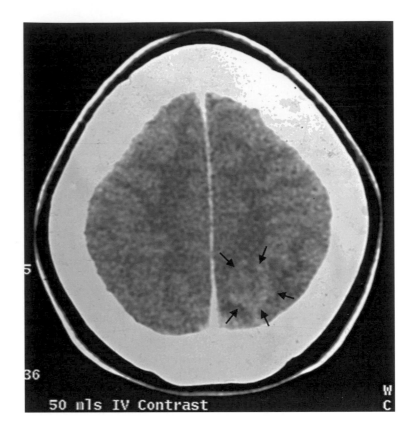

50 nls IV Contrast

13

The angiogram shows (see opposite):
(a) normal flow in the left internal carotid artery;
(b) contrast in the cavernous sinus; this indicates a fistula from (a);
(c) early venous filling.

This is a caroticocavernous fistula. In this case, trauma and a fracture to the base of the skull have caused a tear in the carotid artery at the point of entry into the cavernous sinus. This results in unilateral pulsatile exophthalmos.

Aneurysmal dilatation of the intracavernous portion of the carotid artery anteriorly may result in oedema of the eyelid, exophthalmos, third nerve palsy, pain and loss of vision. Dilatation posteriorly results in pain over the ophthalmic division of the trigeminal nerve and a sixth nerve palsy.

It may be possible in some favourable situations to embolize caroticocavernous fistulae.

13

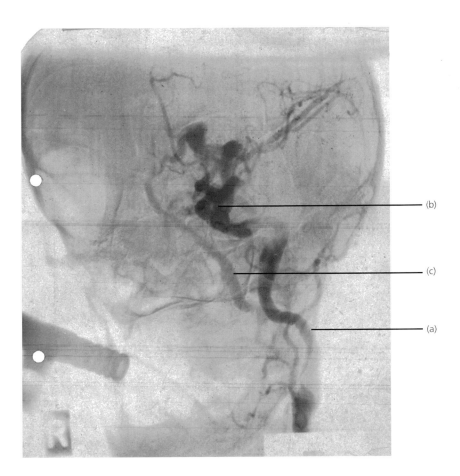

(b)

(c)

(a)

14

The CT scan shows (see overleaf):
(a) low-attenuation changes in the temporal lobe;
(b) low-attenuation changes in the inferior part of the right frontal lobe;
(c) low-attenuation changes in the hippocampus;
(d) a mass effect with midline shift;
(e) central haemorrhage.

An electroencephalogram (EEG) may be useful in showing typical patterns of encephalitis in the region of the temporal lobes.

The diagnosis is herpes simplex encephalitis. This condition can occur at any age, and appears to affect the temporal lobes, possibly due to the spread of reactivated virus from the trigeminal ganglion. Symptoms include fever, headache, personality change and symptoms of temporal lobe involvement. Convulsions, motor or sensory deficit usually occur after one week. The CT image shown is almost diagnostic. Due to the

14

severe oedema, lumbar puncture is usually not performed. Occasionally, a brain biopsy may be required. Early diagnosis and treatment are required, as the mortality is around 55% and half the survivors have serious long-term neurological impairment. These patients require intravenous acyclovir, careful rehydration and mannitol to reduce cerebral oedema.

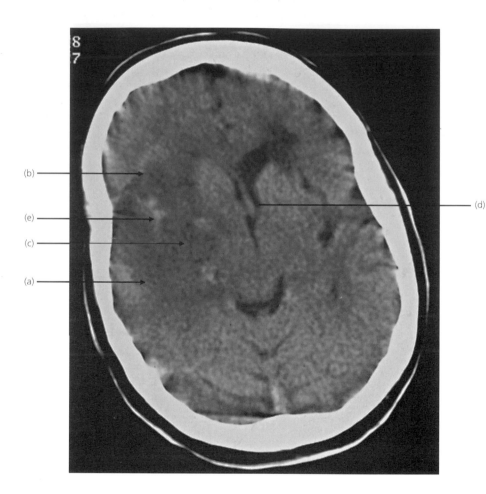

Renal

This is an intravenous urogram which shows:
(a) a horseshoe kidney (shown by arrowheads).

This occurs during embryological development due to fusion of the lower poles of the two kidneys, anterior to the great vessels. Fusion of the upper poles also occurs, but is less common.

The main complications include recurrent infections, ureteric obstruction and the formation of renal calculi. Hydronephrosis is the most common complication, and vesicoureteric reflux is the most important pathological feature. Horseshoe kidneys are a feature of Turner's syndrome.

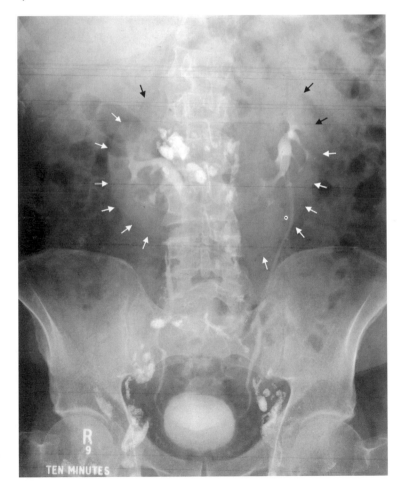

2

The US scan shows:
(a) multiple renal cysts;
(b) multiple cysts in the liver.

The diagnosis is adult polycystic kidney disease (adult PKD). This condition is an inherited autosomal dominant condition, and presents insidiously in middle life, with renal impairment. The commonest site for cyst formation other than the kidney is the liver (around 30%, rising to 80%

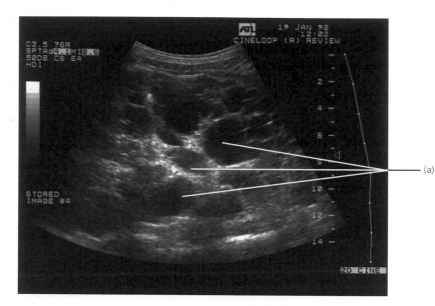

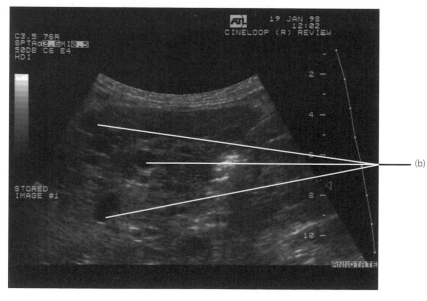

2

after the sixth decade of life). Cysts also occur in the pancreas, spleen, uterus, or ovary.

Renal calculi occur in 10% of patients, leading to pain and haematuria. Care must be taken in these patients, as hypernephromas are more common in adult PKD, and the presence of haematuria should therefore be investigated thoroughly.

Asymptomatic berry aneurysms occur in 7.9% of patients, and rupture of these aneurysms accounted for 6% of deaths in one series. In this group, magnetic resonance angiography (MRA) is recommended every five years, and for recurrent rupture every two or three years. Patients with a family history of intracerebral aneurysm who are between 18 and 35 years of age should be screened using MRA. If this is negative, the examination should be repeated every five years. However, if the MRA proves positive, then an angiogram is required. If the aneurysm is <6 mm in diameter, then the angiogram is repeated after two years. On the other hand, if the aneurysm is 6 mm or more in diameter, it should be treated.

3

The IVU shows (see overleaf):
(a) calcification and autonephrectomy of the left kidney;
(b) clubbing of the calyces and dilatation of the renal pelvis on the right side, consistent with hydronephrosis of the right kidney.

The cause of the renal impairment is renal TB, resulting in autonephrectomy of the left kidney and an obstructive nephropathy on the right, probably secondary to a ureteric stricture.

TB of the renal tract occurs after primary respiratory infection. Usually, the focus of infection is the cortex, with later spread to the papillae. Caseation and discharge into the urine occurs, and may result in a sterile pyuria. Healing usually occurs with the formation of ureteric strictures. An obstructive uropathy usually follows, and calcified caseous material replaces normal renal architecture, i.e. leading to tuberculous autonephrectomy.

Patients require standard anti-TB therapy for six months, with the possible addition of corticosteroids specifically to avoid ureteric stricture formation. Rifampicin, isoniazid and pyrazinamide are given for two months, with rifampicin and isoniazid continuing for four months afterwards. This gives a near-100% cure rate. Corticosteroids are also of value in preserving renal function in tuberculous interstitial nephritis. Surgery to the non-functioning kidney may also be required in cases of severe pain, or if a loin abscess occurs. Surgery does not obviate the need for chemotherapy.

3

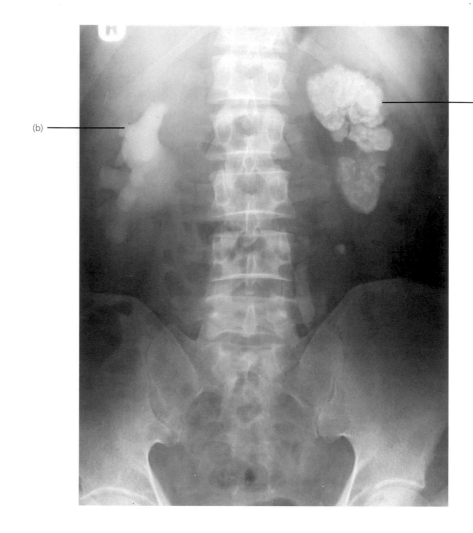

4

These are renal angiograms, which show (see opposite):
(a) multiple intrarenal microaneurysms;
(b) renal cortical infarcts (shown by arrowheads).

The follow-up angiogram was done after a course of pulsed cyclophosphamide, and shows resolution of the microaneurysms as well as:
(c) persistent scarring from the cortical infarcts (shown by arrowheads, see p. 284).

The diagnosis is polyarteritis nodosa (PAN). The stroke may have occurred as a result of cerebral vasculitis, or as a result of renovascular hypertension secondary to PAN.
    PAN is one of the many vasculitides. It affects mainly medium-sized

4

blood vessels, leading to fibrinoid change in the walls and intraluminal thrombus formation. Patients may present with mesenteric, splenic, myocardial, or cerebral infarcts. Repeated renal infarcts lead to hypertension. The diagnosis is confirmed by selective angiography, or a positive perinuclear antineutrophil cytoplasmic antibody (p-ANCA) test (10%), or tissue biopsy. Typical laboratory findings are an increased ESR, increased C-reactive protein (CRP), abnormal LFTs, and renal function. Some patients have positive serology for hepatitis B virus, and these patients respond to interferon-α. Without treatment, the one-year mortality is over 50%. However, with appropriate treatment, the five-year survival rate is more than 80%. Treatment is with cyclophosphamide, methylprednisolone and plasma exchange.

Neurological sequelae occur in around 70% of affected patients. In addition to strokes, these include mononeuritis multiplex, sensorimotor polyneuropathy, fits and psychosis.

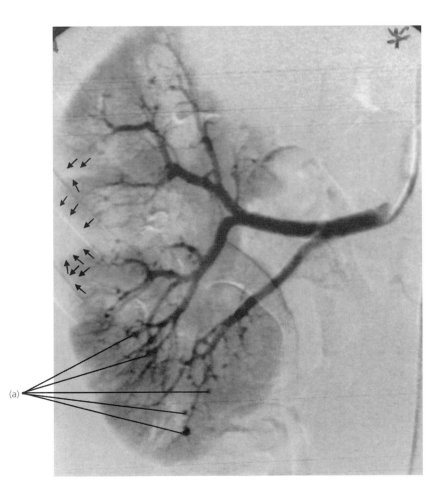

4

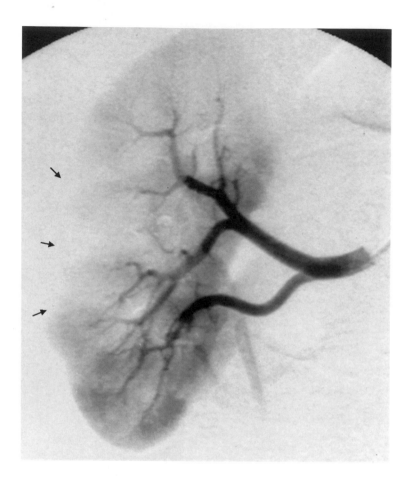

5

The plain abdominal X-ray shows (see opposite):
(a) staghorn calculi.

In this case, the likely cause is hypercalcaemia secondary to sarcoidosis. Nephrocalcinosis occurs in 10% of patients with sarcoidosis.

Renal calculi per se occur in 1–5% of people. They are especially common in warmer climates. The commonest forms contain calcium oxalate alone, or along with calcium phosphate and hydroxyapatite. Other stones are made up of cystine or uric acid. Hypercalciuria is present in 20–40% of patients with calcium-containing stones. Some of these patients also have hypercalcaemia, as in sarcoidosis, hyperparathyroidism, myeloma and malignancy.

Patients usually present with haematuria, loin pain or urinary tract infection (UTI). Small stones of less than 5 mm usually pass spontaneously. Percutaneous nephrolithotomy (PCNL) and extracorporeal shock-wave lithotripsy (ESWL) are suitable for almost all large stones. Open surgery is reserved for urodynamic disorders and staghorn calculi.

5

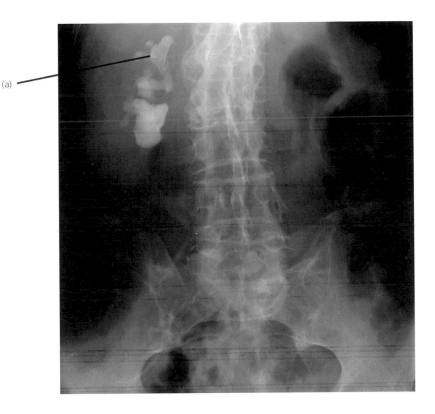

(a)

6

The angiogram shows (see overleaf):
(a) a mass occupying most of the lower pole of the left kidney (shown by arrowheads);
(b) an abnormally rich vascular supply to the lower pole, which is typical of a tumour circulation.

The diagnosis is hypernephroma. Hypernephromas originate from the tubular epithelium, and occur most commonly between the fifth and seventh decades of life. Some 64% of patients present with painless haematuria. Other findings are abdominal mass (25%), loin pain (48%), hypertension (13%), elevated ESR (40%), weight loss, fever and hypercalcaemia; erythrocytosis (3%) due to excess erythropoietin is also seen.

This tumour frequently metastasizes to bone, liver, lung and brain. Useful tests therefore include bone scans, US or CT abdomens.

In the absence of metastases, there is a 65% five-year survival rate after surgery. Tumour staging is the most important single prognostic factor. The hypercalcaemia may be due to metastases, and a bone scan is therefore necessary; or it may be due to a paraneoplastic syndrome, with

6

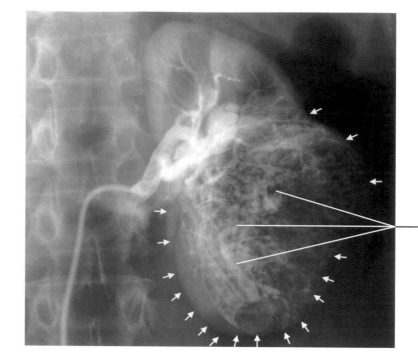

(b)

the production of PTH-related peptide, and therefore unrelated to any osteolytic lesions.

This man may have excess production of erythropoietin, and we would therefore expect him to have a true polycythaemia (1.8–6.0% of patients).

7

The IVU shows (*see opposite*):
Bladder outflow obstruction leading to:
(a) bilateral hydronephrosis with dilation of the pelvis and blunting of the calyces;
(b) bilateral hydroureters.

The abdominal spine X-ray shows (*see p. 288*):
(c) multiple sclerotic metastatic lesions.

The diagnosis is metastatic carcinoma of the prostate, and the back pain is caused by metastatic deposits in the spine. A radioisotope bone scan would be useful to confirm other sites of bony metastasis. The chronic outflow obstruction needs to be relieved in order to prevent progressive renal failure. Initial catheterization and maintenance of correct fluid

7

balance may well correct the renal impairment, but transurethral resection of the prostate (TURP) or open prostatectomy will have to be undertaken in the long run. In some cases, radical prostatectomy with radical radiotherapy may be required. The metastatic deposits in the spine should be treated with adequate analgesia and radiotherapy. Prostatic cancers are dependent on androgens, and this growth factor can therefore be blocked by a specific antagonist, cyproterone acetate. Other alternatives are the use of long-acting luteinizing hormone-releasing hormone (LHRH) analogues, which block pituitary receptors and thus produce a chemical castration by inhibiting testicular stimulation. This should only be used after pretreatment with cyproterone acetate, as the initial surge of luteinizing hormone (LH) will produce a surge of testosterone, causing initial rapid tumour expansion.

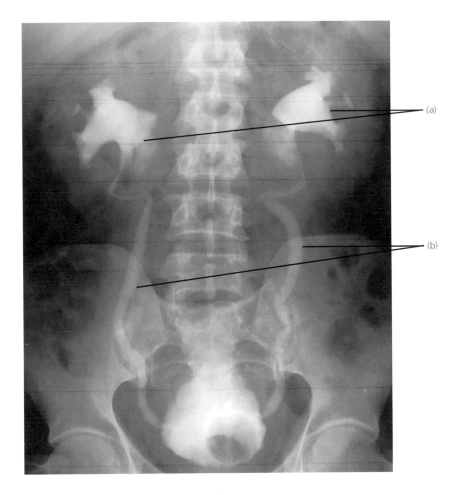

(a)

(b)

7

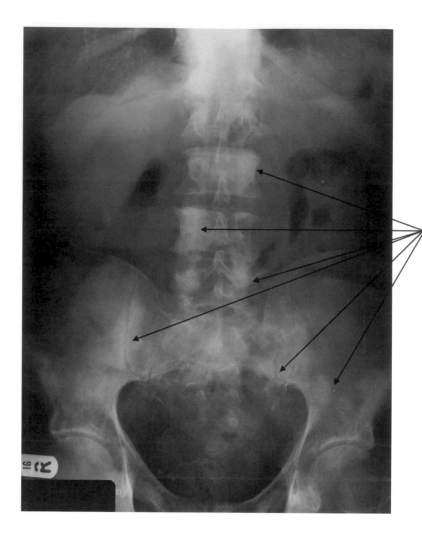

(c)

8

The abdominal X-ray shows (see opposite):
(a) renal calcification;
(b) calculi in the right ureter.

This is typical of medullary sponge kidney. An alternative diagnosis could be renal tubular acidosis (RTA), or renal TB. There is a congenital ectasia of the distal collecting tubule, with enlargement of the pyramids. There is no clear inheritance. The prevalence of this condition is one in 20 000 of the population. It occurs mostly in people between the ages of 20 and 45. The pathology is confined to the medulla. The tubules are dilated, with numerous small cysts. This in turn may lead to RTA and hypercalciuria, which in turn leads to the typical radiological appearance. Patients are often asymptomatic, but others present with UTIs and

8

nephrolithiasis. Microscopic haematuria is almost universal, and proteinuria may also be present. Clinically, medullary sponge kidney is associated with Ehlers–Danlos syndrome and Marfan's syndrome.

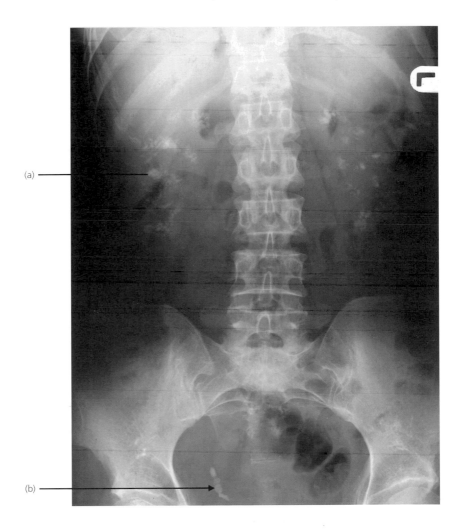

9

This is an angiogram, which shows (see overleaf):
(a) narrowing and severe stenosis of the left renal artery (shown by arrowheads).

The diagnosis is unilateral renal artery stenosis. This has led to renovascular hypertension. The unilateral stenosis leads to a reduction in the pressure in the afferent arterioles of the glomeruli, which is detected by the juxtaglomerular apparatus, and leads to increased renin production. In turn, this leads to an increase in the circulating levels of angiotensin II, which maintains the perfusion of the affected kidney. Renin–angiotensin

9

system (RAS) blockade with angiotensin-converting enzyme (ACE) inhibitors or angiotensin II blockers in this situation leads to marked deterioration in the function of the affected kidney.

There are two main pathological processes: firstly, atherosclerotic disease, which makes up around 75% of cases, and is more common in the elderly. Secondly, there is the familial variety, which is due to fibro-

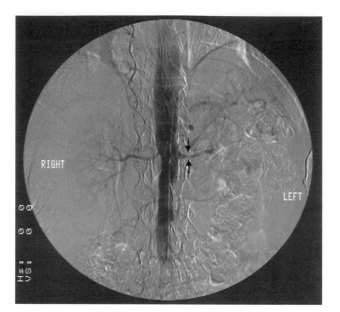

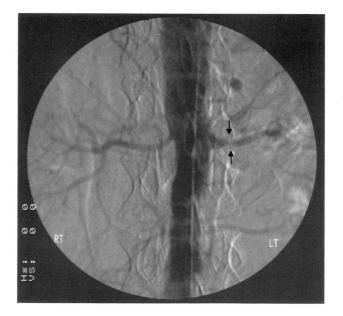

9

muscular hyperplasia and is found more commonly in women; this makes up the remainder of the cases. This variety appears to be associated with an increased incidence of neurofibroma and cerebral aneurysms. The fibromuscular group respond best to balloon angioplasty for middle and distal lesions, and to reconstructive surgery for very proximal and ostial lesions.

10

This is a micturating cystourethrogram, which shows:
(a) bilateral vesicoureteric reflux;
(b) dilatation of the pelvicalyceal system;
(c) clubbing of the calyces.

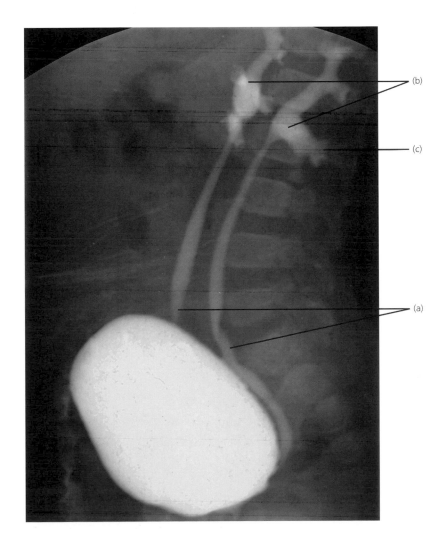

10

The loin pain is due to recurrent episodes of pyelonephritis. The hypertension is due to chronic reflux, leading to bilateral chronic pyelonephritis.

Reflux can be graded into five groups. Grade I represents reflux to the mid-ureter only. Grade II represents reflux to the pelvicalyceal system, but with no dilatation. Grade III is mild to moderate reflux, leading to dilatation and/or tortuosity of the ureters, and mild or moderate dilatation of the pelvis. Grade IV is grade III reflux plus complete obliteration of the sharp angles of the fornices, but with no disturbance of the papillary impressions. Grade V reflux has gross dilatation and tortuosity of the ureters, pelvis and calyces, and the papillary impressions are no longer visible. Reflux is especially common in girls in childhood. They present with recurrent UTIs early in life, or with hypertension or chronic renal failure later. Early surgical correction reduces the risk of developing chronic renal failure.

11

This IVU demonstrates (see below and opposite):
(a) bilateral duplex ureters.

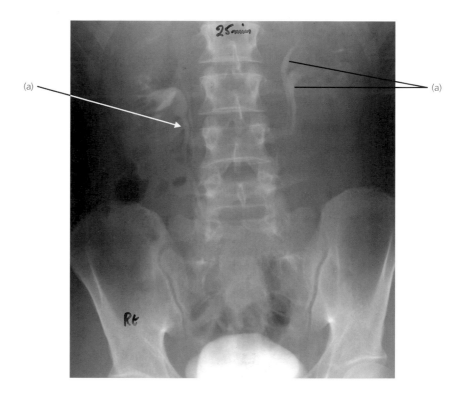

(a)

(a)

11 The upper renal moiety drains into the bladder, but occasionally it may drain into the urethra or vagina in women. This may lead to incontinence or reflux, and there is often obstruction. Recurrent infections lead to scarring of the upper portion and possible hypertension in later years. In some cases, surgical removal of the affected segment is required.

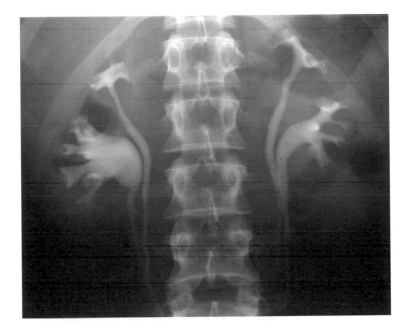

12 *This is a fistulogram. It shows*:
(a) stricture in the fistula.

This is the reason for the patient's inability to dialyse.

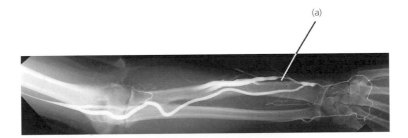

(a)

13

The CT scan of the abdomen shows:
(a) a large renal tumour of the right kidney (shown by arrowheads);
(b) multiple lung metastases.

This is metastatic cancer of the kidney. In view of the lung metastases, surgery is of little benefit. The patient could be referred for palliative chemotherapy. The results of embolization, chemotherapy and hormone therapy have been disappointing. However, immunotherapy using lymphokine-activated killer cells combined with recombinant IL-2 has shown some benefit in tumour suppression.

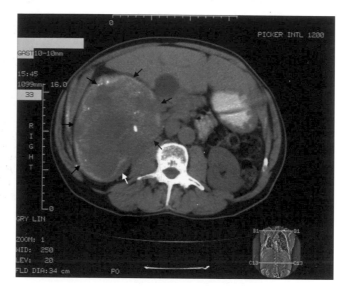

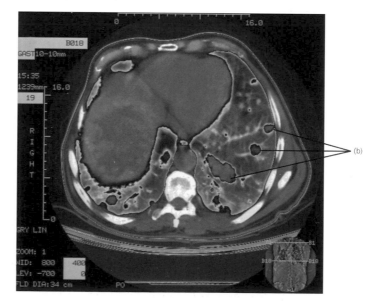

Respiratory Medicine

1

This chest X-ray shows:
(a) multiple calcified foci.

This is typical of old healed previous varicella zoster pneumonitis. In addition, it may be noted that there is also upper lobe diversion.

   Varicella zoster pneumonitis may be a component of primary infection, i.e. chickenpox, and should not be confused with reactivation (shingles). This is usually a self-limiting condition, but the acute phase can be fatal especially in adults. It may present with chest pain, shortness of breath, pulmonary oedema and cyanosis. The evidence for previous infection are the diffuse calcified lesions, which may be mistaken for miliary TB.

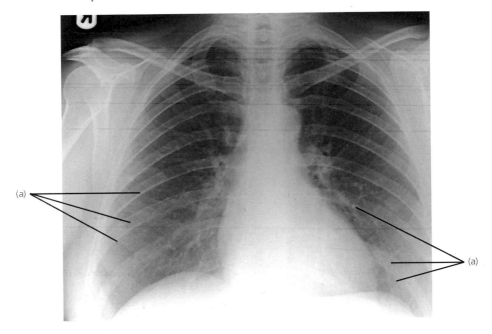

2

This is a bronchogram (see overleaf), which is produced by the injection of dye into the trachea or bronchi via a naso tracheal tube or now, more usually, selectively via a bronchoscope, resulting in the image shown.

The bronchogram shows:
(a) distortion and dilatation of the bronchi, giving rise to:
(b) the appearance of ring shadows;
(c) or line shadows 1–2 cm in diameter.

2

In asthma, mucus plugging together with immunological inflammation leads to secondary infection and collapse. This subsequently leads to thinning and dilatation of the bronchial walls. Differential diagnoses include Kartagener's syndrome and cystic fibrosis.

The haemoptysis is secondary to bronchiectasis. *Aspergillus* is a common organism in asthmatics, and recurrent infections may lead to bronchiectasis. Aspergillomas, and not bronchopulmonary aspergillosis, give rise to haemoptysis. Current *Aspergillus* infection can be diagnosed by a positive skin-prick test, venous sampling for *Aspergillus* precipitins, and sputum culture either directly or from bronchial washings, to look for invasive fungal hyphae. Bronchograms are used infrequently, and this test has been largely superseded by high-resolution CT.

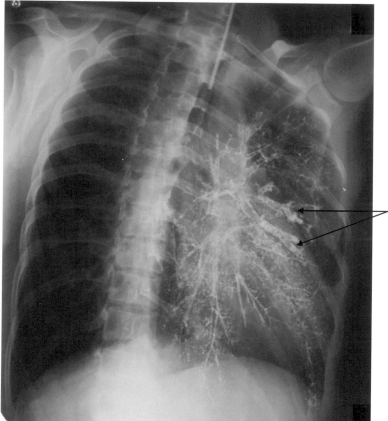

Bronchiecta

3

The CXR shows (see opposite and p. 298):
(a) hyperinflation of both lungs;
(b) tramline appearance in the left lung;
(c) ring shadow vascular markings in both lungs.

3

These features are characteristic of diffuse bronchiectasis. These changes are seen most commonly in the upper lobes.

The diagnosis is cystic fibrosis, which can be confirmed by the sodium sweat test, which involves measurement of sodium in sweat by iontophoresis after the administration of pilocarpine. Two values >60 mmol/L confirm the diagnosis.

Cystic fibrosis presents in the neonatal period with meconium ileus, due to the thick viscid secretions. Together with pancreatic insufficiency, this leads to malabsorption, and 80% of patients develop intussusception or intestinal obstruction. Portal hypertension, pneumothorax and cor pulmonale are also common. Fifty per cent of patients have diabetes mellitus. Respiratory tract infections are common, usually resulting from *Staphylococcal* or *Pseudomonas* infections. Treatment is by mucolytics, physiotherapy, postural drainage and aggressive treatment of infections. End-stage management includes referral for heart/lung transplantation.

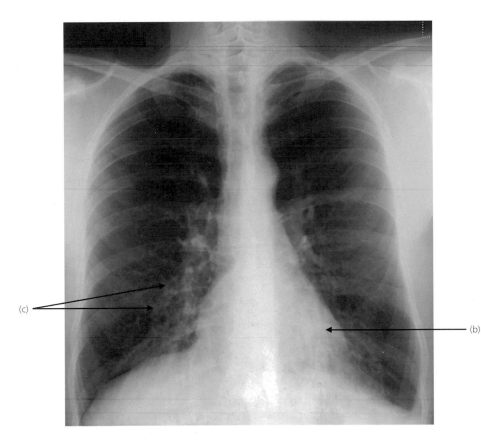

3

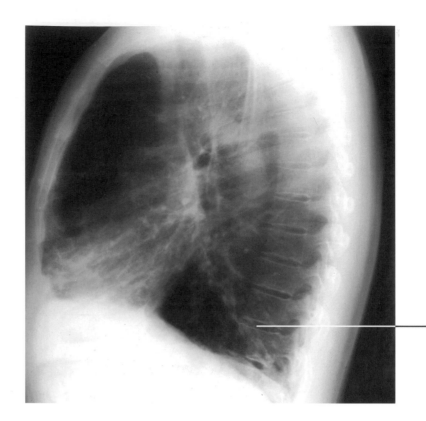

(b)

4   *The CXR shows (see opposite top)*:
(a) unilateral hypertranslucency of the right lung;
(b) reduction in right-sided hilar markings;
(c) reduced peripheral vascular markings in the right lung field;
(d) mediastinal shift to the right.

The diagnosis is MacLeod's syndrome. A pulmonary angiogram showing the absence of a right pulmonary artery, or a V/Q scan showing reduced ventilation and perfusion of the right lung, would help support the above diagnosis.

A viral obliterative bronchiolitis in children leads to hypoplasia of the lung, with a reduction in the number of alveoli and a small pulmonary artery. The infection occurs during the active phase of lung growth. Most patients are asymptomatic, but some may present with chronic bronchitis and a mild obstructive defect. The CXR *(see opposite bottom)* shows the same abnormality in an infant.

4

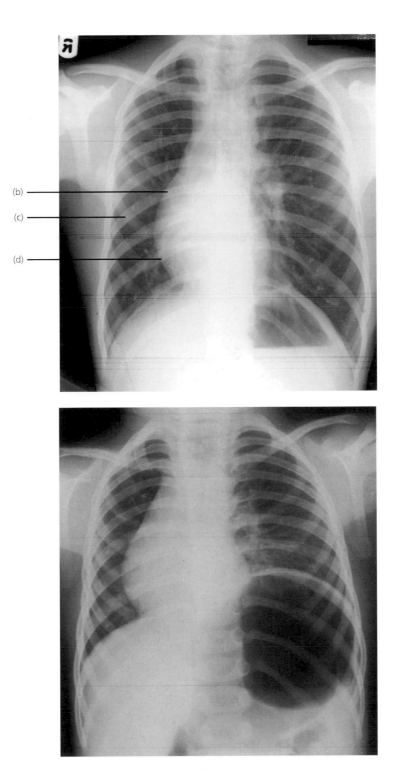

(b)

(c)

(d)

5

The CXR shows:
(a) right apical shadowing;
(b) destruction of the second rib.

The diagnosis is a Pancoast tumour (pulmonary sulcus tumor).

Associated features may include Horner's syndrome due to involvement of the inferior cervical sympathetic ganglion, wasting of the small muscles of the hand if the brachial plexus becomes involved, and rarely cord compression. In the case of a left-sided Pancoast tumour, vocal cord paralysis may occur if the left recurrent laryngeal nerve is involved.

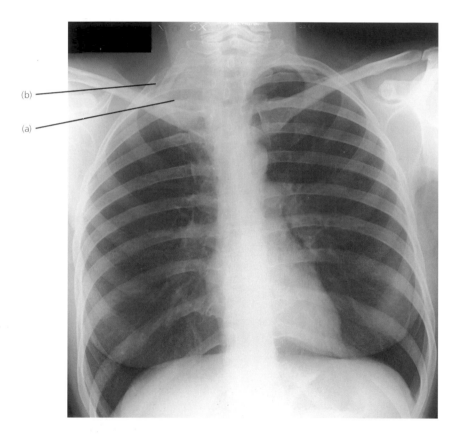

6

The CXR shows (see opposite):
(a) an opacity in the left upper zone, within
(b) a thick-walled cavity (shown by arrowheads).

The diagnosis is an aspergilloma in an old tuberculous cavity. The diagnosis can be confirmed by sputum cultures for *Aspergillus*, or by confirming raised antibody titres to *Aspergillus*. Aspergillomas can be removed surgically, or alternatively can be embolized. Antifungal treatment alone is rarely effective.

6

Around 15% of people with tuberculous cavities have radiological evidence of aspergillosis, and of these another 10% develop life-threatening haemoptysis. One-third of patients with aspergillosis are serum-positive for *Aspergillus*. The presentation is usually with cough or haemoptysis. In severe or invasive cases surgical removal should be considered, provided lung function tests are satisfactory.

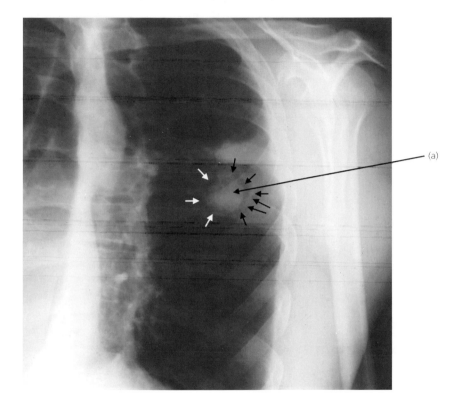

(a)

7

The CXR shows (see overleaf top):
(a) bilateral hilar lymphadenopathy.

Other features that can occur are (*see overleaf bottom*):
(b) fibrosis in both lung fields;
(c) eggshell calcification of the hila (not shown here);
(d) or calcification within the hila itself, as shown in the X-ray of a different patient.

The hand X-ray shows (see p. 303):
(e) multiple bone cysts in a lace-like pattern.

The diagnosis is sarcoidosis. This can be confirmed by transbronchial biopsy, open lung biopsy, liver or bone marrow biopsy, the measurement

7

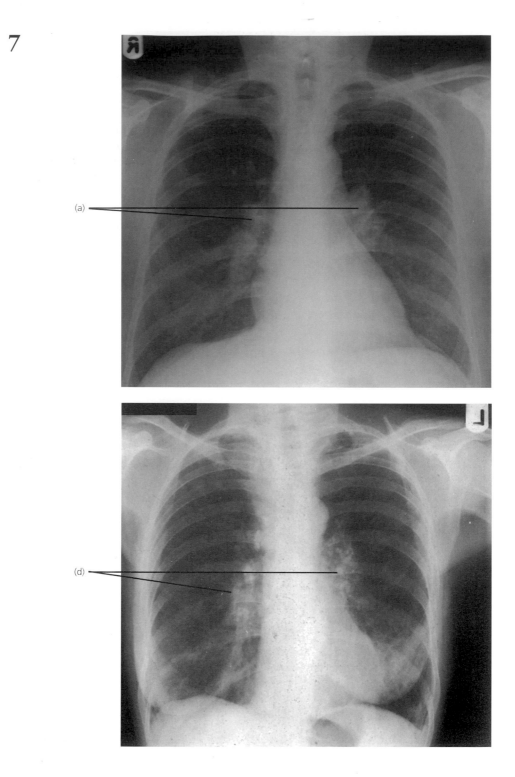

(a)

(d)

7

of serum ACE levels, and a positive Kveim test. A negative tuberculin test would provide supportive evidence, but would not confirm the diagnosis. The combination of sarcoidosis with enlargement of the parotid glands, fever and uveitis is known as Heerfordt's syndrome.

Sarcoidosis is a granulomatous disease that commonly affects the respiratory tract. There are three common presentations, with very different prognoses. Firstly, there is bilateral hilar lymphadenopathy (BHL), which is self-remitting in 80% of cases. The next stage is BHL with pulmonary infiltrates, which remits in 40% of cases. Finally, there may be marked pulmonary fibrosis with severe restrictive lung defects; this may carry the worst prognosis, as conventional immunosuppressive regimens with steroids and azathioprine may be of little value. The skin may be involved, with lupus pernio and erythema nodosum. The eyes are also involved, with a painful anterior uveitis or reduced visual acuity in posterior uveitis. Bone cysts and parotid gland and lacrimal gland enlargement also occur. Hypercalcaemia due to increased production of vitamin D within the granulomas is common, and may lead to renal failure.

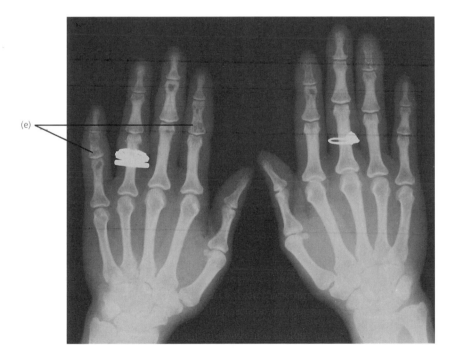

8

The CXR shows (see overleaf):
(a) a solitary pulmonary nodule (shown by arrowheads).

The likely diagnosis is a neurofibroma or other neurogenic tumour, or a hamartoma. A benign tumour is more likely in a completely asympto-

8

matic individual. In general, primary lung malignancy becomes more probable after the age of 45, in males and smokers. Lesions are usually greater than 2 cm in diameter, lack calcification and have ill-defined, spiculated margins. Secondary tumours may be much smaller than 2 cm, and the above criteria do not apply to these.

Other benign lesions are tuberculomas, hydatid cysts, histoplasmosis, or pulmonary infarcts. Approximately 80% of nodules in the lung are due to carcinoma, 10% are due to other tumours and the remaining 10% are made up of the above causes.

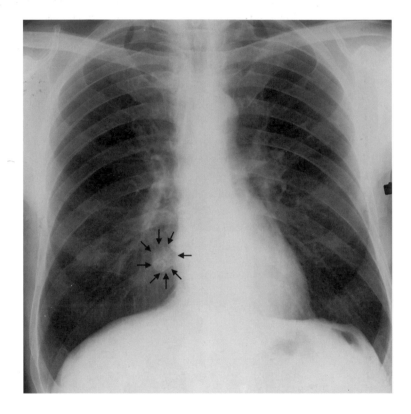

9

The CXR shows (see opposite):
(a) a cavity in the left lung field (shown by arrowheads);
(b) containing a fluid level.

This is an abscess in a lung cavity.

The likely diagnosis is bacterial endocarditis of the tricuspid valve, with resultant septic embolization to the lung and the development of an abscess-containing cavity. Usually these are multiple. Echocardiography will help confirm endocarditis of the tricuspid valve, and blood cultures

9

and sputum cultures may help determine the organism. Intravenous drug abusers are at high risk of staphylococcal endocarditis, with the tricuspid valve being the commonest site of infection. If embolization to the lung occurs, single or multiple infected pulmonary infarcts result, and ultimately abscess formation may develop. Abscess formation may also occur as a result of direct haematogenous spread. Specific causes of infection lead to characteristic sites of abscess formation. Amoebic or subphrenic abscess may lead to secondary abscess formation in the right lower lobe. Although the right lower lobe is the commonest site for aspiration in the upright patient, the posterior segment of the right upper lobe is the common site following aspiration, due to oesophageal obstruction whilst supine. Bronchial obstruction anywhere may lead to distal abscess formation from resolving *Staphylococcal, Klebsiella* or *Streptococcus milleri* infection.

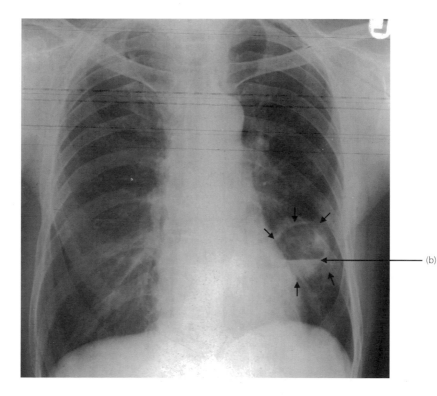

(b)

10

The CXR shows (*see overleaf*):
(a) a large soft-tissue mass involving the right pleura;
(b) a pleural effusion;
(c) destruction of the ribs;
(d) pleural calcification.

10

Other features which may be seen (not shown here) are:
(e) extensive pleural plaques;
(f) pulmonary fibrosis.

The diagnosis in this man is a mesothelioma of the right lung. During his working life, he was probably exposed to asbestos. Exposure to asbestos fibres can lead to pulmonary fibrosis and the formation of pleural plaques in a dose-dependent manner. Crocidolite (blue) and amosite (brown) are more strongly associated with mesothelioma than chrysotile (white). The risk of lung cancer following exposure is additive to the effect of smoking. Industries typically associated with this are the ship-building industry, fireproofing (clothes or insulation), car industry (bonding of brake lining) and lagging.

Pleural plaques may be found incidentally in people living near manufacturers in these industries. In these cases, they are of no further significance.

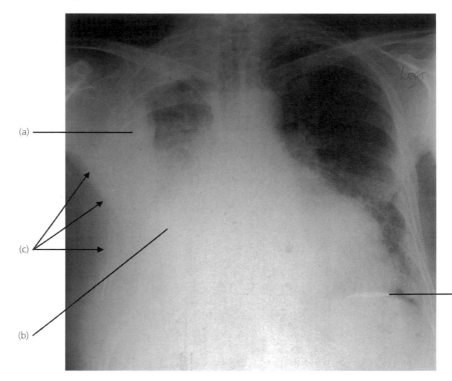

11

The CXR shows (see opposite):
(a) round opacities in the upper zone and mid-zone, which coalesce and occupy around one-third of the lung (shown by arrowheads);
(b) fibrosis.

11

Occasionally, the CXR shows:
(c) cavitation;
(d) rheumatoid nodules (Kaplan's syndrome).

This man presented with coal miner's pneumoconiosis, but has now developed end-stage progressive massive fibrosis.

Inhaled coal dust is phagocytosed by macrophages, which in turn release a number of cytotoxic products that lead to fibrosis and destruction of the lymph node. Coal dust itself may directly stimulate a fibrotic reaction. Simple pneumoconiosis has few signs, and radiologically appears as upper zone fibrosis. It may spread to the rest of the lung and coalesce to develop progressive massive fibrosis. These patients are extremely short of breath and there is melanoptysis, which is expectoration of the black contents of the cavitating lung lesions.

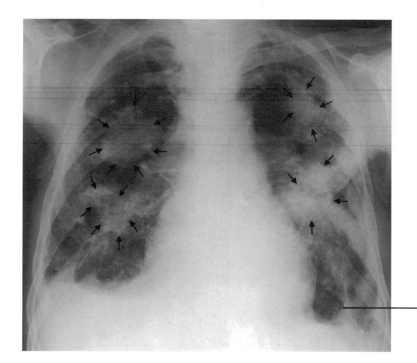

(b)

12

The CXR shows (see overleaf):
(a) multiple pulmonary opacities, which appear to be cavitating (shown by arrowheads). These radiological changes often come and go, and;
may represent disease activity. Pulmonary haemorrhage may give rise to haemosiderosis and;
(b) residual miliary calcification.

12

The diagnosis is Wegener's granulomatosis. Serum testing for cytoplasmic antineutrophil cytoplasmic antibody (c-ANCA) and a renal biopsy would help confirm the diagnosis.

This is a vasculitic disease, and commonly affects the glomeruli and the upper and lower respiratory tracts. It may affect other areas, such as heart valves and the central nervous system. Patients may present with cough haemoptysis and occasionally chest pain. Radiologically, there may be nodules, cavities and flitting reticulonodular shadows. Occasionally, pneumothoraces or pleural effusions occur as a result of the condition. The renal lesion is a focal necrotizing glomerulonephritis. Death usually occurs as a result of renal disease. Previously, these patients were treated with steroids. However, the use of cyclophosphamide has improved the prognosis considerably.

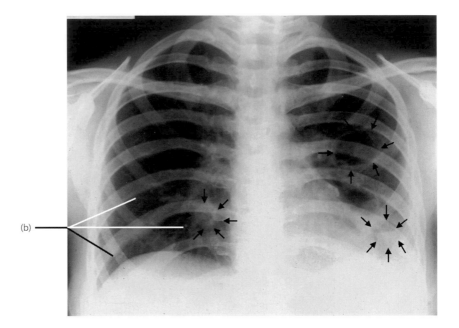

13

The CXR shows (see opposite top):
(a) loss of the left hemidiaphragm silhouette;
(b) a shadow next to the left heart border of intermediate density to lung and heart tissue;
(c) displacement of the left hilum towards the diaphragm;
(d) tracheal deviation to the left.

These features represent collapse of the left lower lobe. Collapse of the lobe results in mediastinal shift and tracheal deviation towards the side of the lesion. The hilum is also displaced inferiorly. Loss of air in the

13

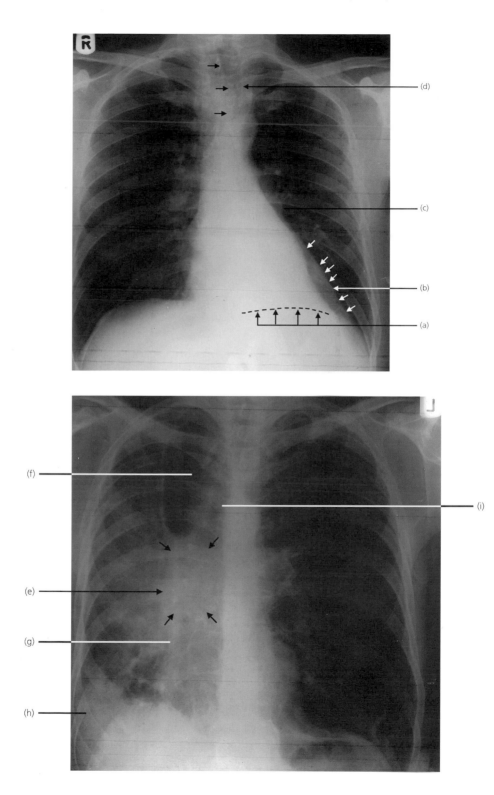

13   lower lobe results in tissue of similar radiopacity lying adjacent to the left heart border and the left hemidiaphragm. This results in a loss of the typical silhouette.

The CXR (*see p. 309 bottom*) shows a similar situation on the right side, with collapse of the right middle and lower lobes. It shows:
(e) a large right hilar mass;
(f) mediastinal shift to the right;
(g) loss of the right heart border—right middle lobe (RML) collapse;
(h) loss of the right hemidiaphragm silhouette—right lower lobe (RLL) collapse;
(i) tracheal deviation to the right.

14   *The CXR shows (see below):*
(a) a large shadow in the right upper zone with ill-defined margins;
(b) an enlarged mediastinum (shown by arrowheads).

The venogram of the upper limb shows (see opposite):
(a) sudden cessation of contrast media in the superior vena cava;
(b) dilatation of the venous drainage of the upper limbs;
(c) increase in collateral flow in the superficial veins towards the inferior vena cava;
(d) retrograde filling of the azygos and hemiazygos veins.

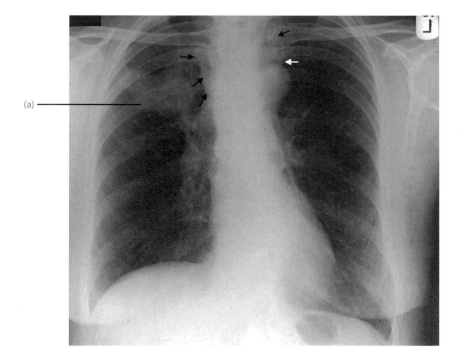

(a)

14

The diagnosis is superior vena caval obstruction. The cause in this case is carcinoma of the lung (75%). Other causes include lymphoma, aortic aneurysm and retrosternal goitre. Patients present with facial and upper limb oedema. Headaches are also a common symptom. In this case, radiotherapy was used to shrink the tumour mass and relieve the obstruction.

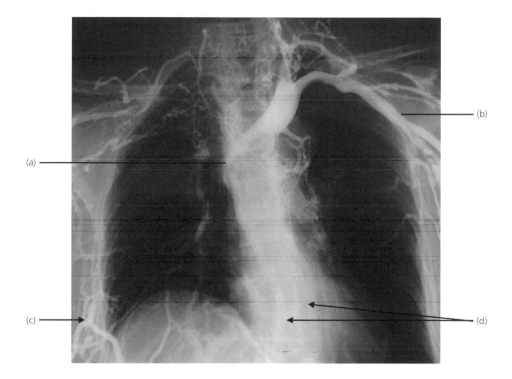

15

The CXR shows (see overleaf):
(a) mass in the anterior mediastinum (shown by arrowheads).

In the clinical scenario given, the likely diagnosis is a thymoma. The patient is suffering from myasthenia gravis. Without a clinical history, the differential diagnosis includes lymphadenopathy, a retrosternal thyroid or a dermoid tumour.

The diagnosis can be confirmed by the Tensilon test, and demonstrates fatigability of a group of muscles, which can be reversed by short-acting acetylcholinesterase inhibitors. Alternatively, IgG levels to the acetylcholine (Ach) receptor is positive in around 90% of cases. Other muscle groups affected are the extraocular muscles; the bulbar group, resulting in dysphagia; the intercostal group, resulting in dyspnoea; and the proximal skeletal muscles. This condition can be treated with

15

immunosuppression, with drugs such as prednisolone and azathioprine, as well as acetylcholinesterase inhibitors such as neostigmine. Plasmapheresis may also be undertaken to reduce circulating antibodies to the acetylcholine receptor. Thymomas are more common in women and in the young. In cases associated with a thymoma, thymectomy may cure or greatly improve the severity of the myasthenia.

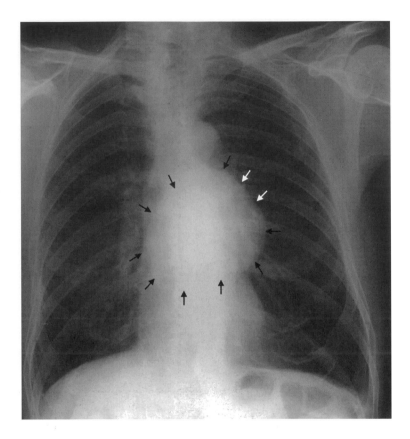

16

The CXR shows (*see opposite*):
(a) surgical emphysema;
(b) a left pneumothorax;
(c) pneumopericardium (double heart border);
(d) pneumomediastinum.

The dramatic radiological appearance is due to a ruptured bronchus, which results in mediastinal emphysema. If the air subsequently escapes to the subcutaneous tissues, this results in surgical emphysema.

16

Coarse crepitations can be heard over the precordium, as well as a loud systolic crunch due to the presence of the left-sided pneumothorax. This is known as Hamman's sign.

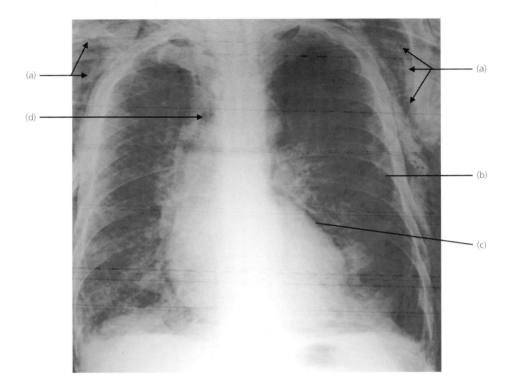

17

The test shown is a ventilation–perfusion scan. It shows (see overleaf):
(a) a large perfusion defect in the lower right lung;
(b) a small perfusion defect in the upper part of the right lung;
(c) multiple perfusion defects in the left lung;
(d) normal ventilation of both lungs.

This test shows a ventilation–perfusion mismatch, and confirms the diagnosis of multiple pulmonary embolism. In view of the patient's young age and history, blood samples should be sent for lupus anticoagulant, anticardiolipin antibody, and antinuclear antibody (ANA) testing. Without her clinical history, a deficiency in proteins S, C and antithrombin III, or a factor V Leiden mutation should also be sought. The latter confers activated protein C resistance, and occurs in 4% of the population. The homozygous form is associated with a seven-fold increase in thromboembolism. The history of arthritis, renal impairment and pul-

17   monary embolus should alert the clinician to the probability of SLE with lupus anticoagulant syndrome. Treatments include anticoagulation, peripheral thrombolysis, intrapulmonary thrombolysis, catheter embolectomy, and surgical embolectomy.

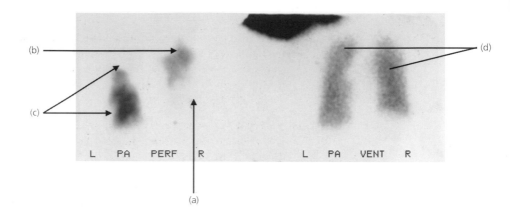

Skeletal

1

The X-ray of the hands shows:
(a) telescoping of the phalanges (the so-called 'opera glass hands');
(b) erosions and bone resorption;
(c) the distal phalanx shows the 'pencil-in-cup' deformity;
(d) bone loss and tapering of the proximal joint surface;
(e) splaying of the distal joint surface.

The diagnosis is arthritis mutilans, or psoriatic arthropathy. This occurs in 8–10% of patients with psoriasis, and may be associated with an extensive skin rash. The cervical spine, lumbar spine, hips and sacroiliac joints may also be involved, in a manner in keeping with spondylo-arthropathy. Other patterns of arthropathy associated with psoriasis include a polyarthritis that mimics rheumatoid arthritis (RhA), but is seronegative. There may be spondylotic changes, as in ankylosing spondylitis, and this pattern of disease is associated with HLA-B27 in around 70% of cases. There is also an asymmetrical oligoarthritis affecting the large joints in the lower limb. However, the most characteristic form involves the distal interphalangeal joint, and is associated with nail changes.

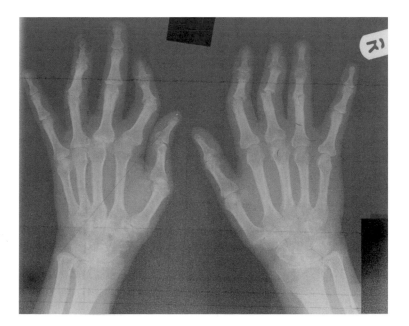

2

The X-ray of the knee shows (see below and opposite):
(a) chondrocalcinosis.

The diagnosis is pyrophosphate arthropathy, or pseudogout. This can be confirmed by aspirating the knee to look for weakly positively birefringent rhomboidal-shaped crystals. These calcium pyrophosphate crystals are deposited in the cartilage, and give rise to the typical radiological appearance described. Although the condition is most commonly idiopathic and age-related, it is associated with hyperparathyroidism, hypothyroidism and haemachromatosis. If clinically suggested, tests for

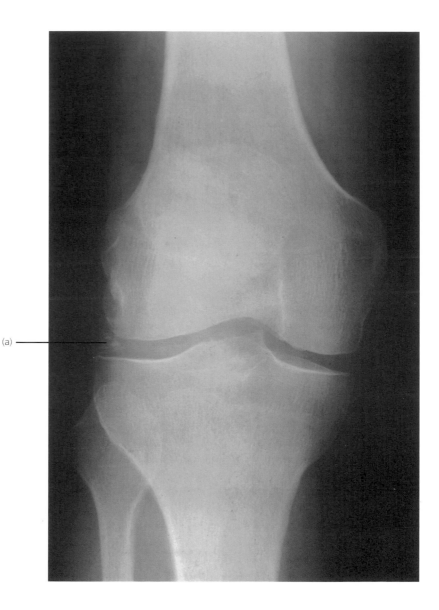

(a) —

2

serum Ca, TSH, Fe, total iron-binding capacity (TIBC), transferrin and ferritin may all therefore be useful here. Management involves treating the primary condition if present, and pain relief with NSAIDs and possibly intra-articular steroid injections. Colchicine may also be useful for acute exacerbations.

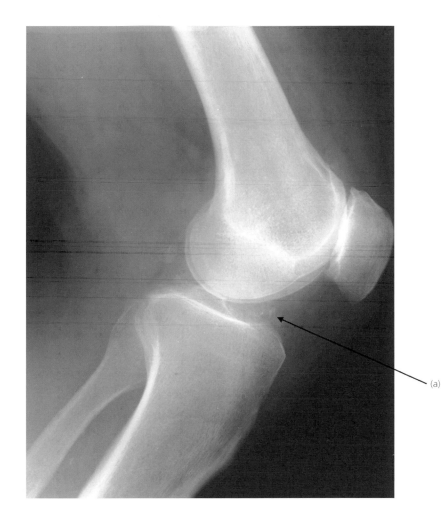

(a)

3

The X-rays show (see overleaf):
(a) calcification (calcinosis) of the soft tissues of the fingertips;
(b) pulp resorption and tapering of the fingers.

The calcification may also be found at other sites, e.g. the knee joint (c) (*see pp. 319 and 320*).

3

This woman may well be complaining of dysphagia due to oesophageal dysmotility, as well as painful hands and feet due to Raynaud's phenomenon.

On inspection, one would expect to find telangiectasia and sclerodactyly. The diagnosis is CREST syndrome or limited scleroderma. Systemic sclerosis is a multisystem disease that leads to progressive fibrosis and atrophy. It may exist in limited or diffuse forms. The female to male ratio is 3:1. The skin becomes thickened and tethered. Raynaud's phenomenon occurs in about 95% of cases, and may lead to digital loss. Myositis, polyarthritis (usually non-destructive), calcinosis and basal pulmonary fibrosis (45% of cases) also occur. Death is usually the result of cardiac involvement, either due to pulmonary hypertension or acute heart failure caused by a hypertensive crisis. Severe bowel involvement may also occur with advanced disease. The CREST syndrome is a milder or limited form and has a better prognosis, although pulmonary hypertension is increasingly recognized. The diagnosis is made clinically, although anticentromere antibodies and the anti-Scl 70 autoantibody may be positive in the CREST syndrome and diffuse systemic sclerosis, respectively. Treatment is symptomatic, with vasodilators and heated gloves for Raynaud's. Active pulmonary involvement is an indication for treatment with cyclophosphamide. Bacterial overgrowth responds to antibiotic therapy, and proton-pump inhibitors are useful for oesophageal disease. ACE inhibition is an effective treatment for hypertension. Normotensive renal crisis may be precipitated by steroid therapy.

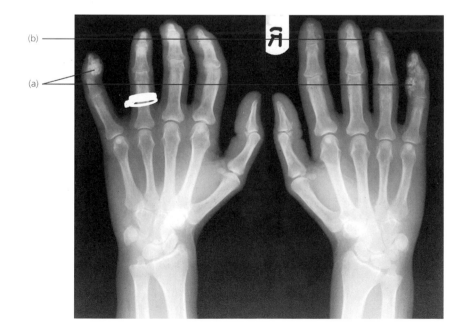

3

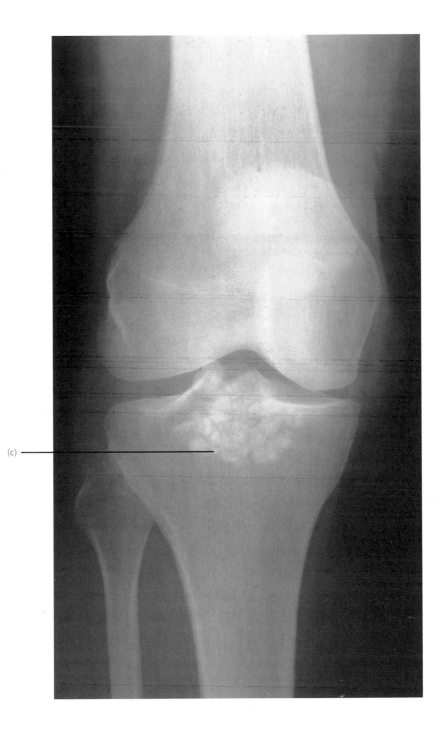

(c) ———————————

3

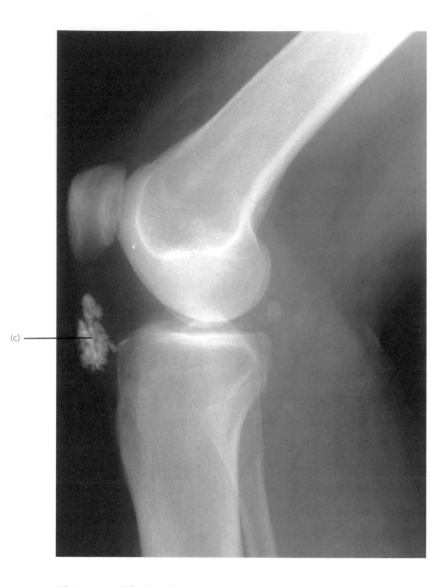

(c) ——

4

The X-ray of the hip shows (opposite top):
(a) osteopenia due to defective bone mineralization;
(b) areas of sclerosis, which are known as Looser's zones or pseudofractures;

The X-ray of the arm shows (opposite bottom):
(c) a Looser's zone on the ulna;
(d) a brown tumour on the humerus (due to hyperparathyroidism).
Looser's zones are also seen on the scapula, pelvis, long bones and ribs.

Other classical areas to become affected are the vertebral bodies as shown on p. 322.
(e) The vertebral bodies may become biconcave, producing the so-called 'codfish spine' appearance.

4

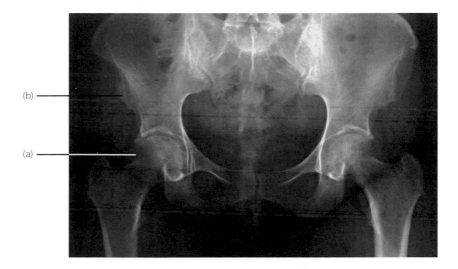

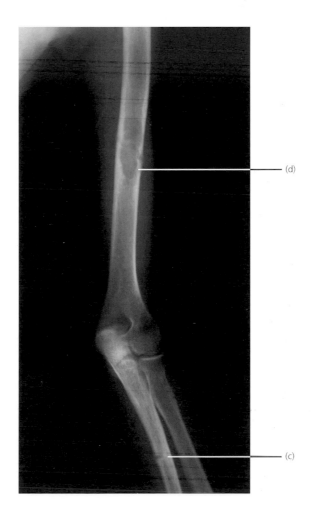

4

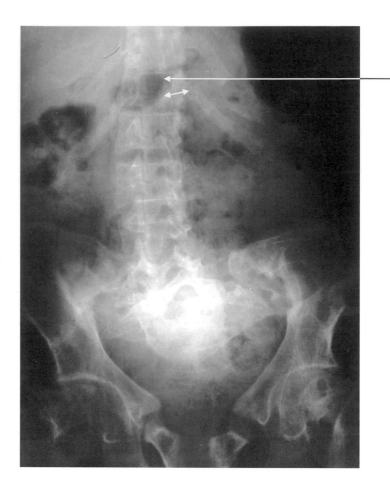

(e)

(f) Later radiological changes of secondary or tertiary hyperparathyroidism may be superimposed.

The diagnosis is osteomalacia secondary to malabsorption. The malabsorption is likely to be due to a gluten-sensitive enteropathy, which is associated with dermatitis herpetiformis.

A jejunal biopsy showing subtotal villous atrophy, which improves when gluten is eliminated from the diet, will help to confirm the diagnosis. Serum Ca and PO_4 will be low, and alkaline phosphatase increased. Antireticulin, antigliadin and antiendomysial antibodies may be positive, supporting the above diagnosis. There may be malabsorption of other important nutrients such as Fe and folic acid. The treatment is to avoid gluten and to treat severe skin lesions with dapsone. Osteomalacia is more common in Asian women residing in the West, partly as a result of dietary deficiencies and partly due to a lifestyle that may keep them indoors, and thus reduce endogenous production of vitamin D.

The walking difficulty caused by a proximal myopathy or hypocalcaemia.

5

The X-ray shows (see below):
(a) demineralization of the vertebral bodies;
(b) simultaneous new bone formation along the subchondral plates.

This is the 'rugger jersey spine' appearance.

The X-ray of the hands show (see overleaf):
(c) resorption of the distal phalanges;
(d) subperiosteal resorption;
(e) the soft tissue swelling at the wrist from the AV fistula.

The diagnosis is renal osteodystrophy. Due to renal disease, there is a failure of the renal hydroxylation of cholecalciferol, which is required to make it metabolically active. This results in poor absorption of Ca from the gut, resulting in low serum Ca and increased PO_4 levels. This in turn leads to secondary hyperparathyroidism, which may then become autonomous and lead to tertiary hyperparathyroidism. Treatment involves the use of aluminium hydroxide gel to lower serum phosphate levels, the use of 1α-OH cholecalciferol to increase serum calcium levels and hence reduce PTH production, and finally parathyroidectomy in cases of tertiary hyperparathyroidism. It should be noted that these gross radiological changes are becoming less common now.

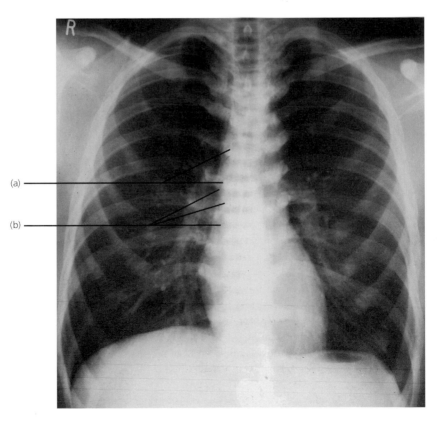

5

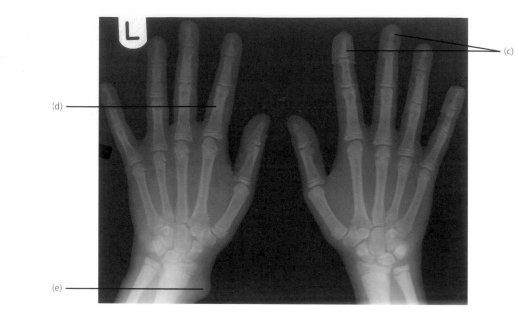

(c)

(d)

(e)

6

The skull X-ray shows (see opposite top):
(a) areas of lucency secondary to bone resorption (osteolysis);
(b) areas of increased bone density, secondary to osteoblastic activity;
(c) gross thickening of the vault.

Bone reabsorption and formation is completely disorganized, giving rise to the above appearance.

The diagnosis is Paget's disease or osteitis deformans, which occurs in around 10% of elderly people. There is increased osteoclastic activity, which is compensated by increased osteoblastic activity, resulting in disorganization of the normal bone architecture and an increase in vascularity. Blindness may occur as a result of nerve compression.

The lateral skull X-ray shows (see opposite bottom):
(d) platybasia with occipital invagination;
(e) enlargement of the skull.

Deafness is a result of compression of the eighth cranial nerve, although occasionally it can be caused by involvement of the ossicles. The skull, axial skeleton and long bones are usually involved, resulting in characteristic deformities such as bowing of the tibia (sabre tibia) (f) (*see p. 326*). Occasionally, there is malignant transformation, and osteosarcomas can occur. Another important cause of mortality is high-output cardiac failure.

6   The serum Ca and PO$_4$ are usually normal, but alkaline phosphatase is increased. Urinary 24-hour hydroxyproline is increased in this condition. There are possible links with canine distemper virus. Treatment may include calcitonin and bisphosphonates to reduce bone turnover.

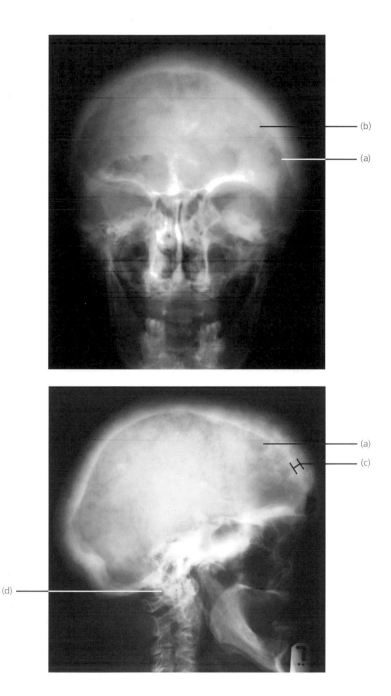

6

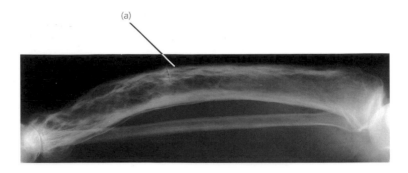

(a)

7

The X-ray shows (see opposite and p. 328):
(a) squaring of the vertebrae due to subperiosteal new bone formation;
(b) erosions at the site of insertion of the annulus fibrosus (Romanus lesions);
(c) formation of syndesmophytes at the margins of the vertebral bodies.

When ankylosis is complete, the appearances are often described as a 'bamboo spine'. Fusion of the sacroiliac joints may also be seen (not shown here).

The diagnosis is ankylosing spondylitis. This condition has a prevalence of 1% and a male to female ratio of 9:1. Around 95% of those affected are HLA-B27 positive. The sacroiliac joints are always involved, resulting in low back pain that radiates to the buttocks. There may also be a loss of the lumbar lordosis and a fixed kyphosis with extension of the cervical spine, giving rise to the appearance known as the 'question-mark spine'.

The shortness of breath may be due to ankylosis of the rib joints leading to reduced chest expansion, or due to aortic regurgitation secondary to aortitis (4% of cases), or may result from pulmonary fibrosis, which appears radiologically at the apices (1.5%).

The electrocardiogram (ECG) may show some form of heart block. Cardiac conduction defects occur in 10% of cases. Another feature is iritis (30%).

7

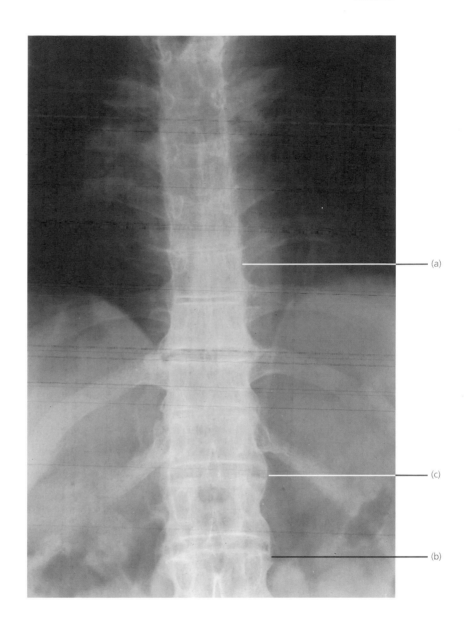

(a)

(c)

(b)

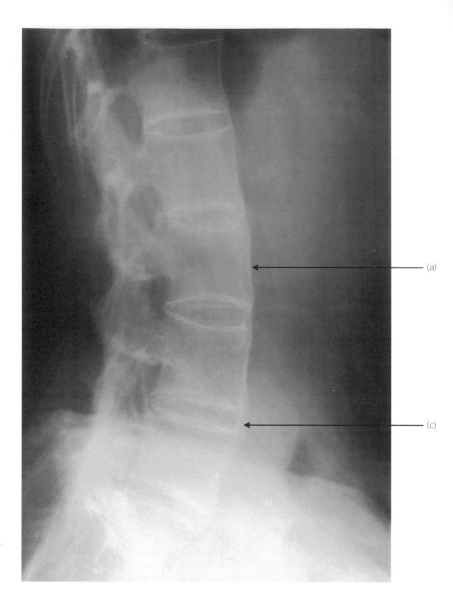

8

The X-ray of the foot shows (see opposite and p. 330):
(a) destruction of the cartilage;
(b) excessive disorganized new bone formation;
(c) subchondral bone fractures;
(d) bone resorption, producing this final appearance, which is typical appearance of a Charcot's joint.

8 Loss of joint position and pain leads to abnormal stress on the joints, which in turn leads to the radiological appearances shown.

A fasting blood glucose and serum for VDRL or TPHA testing would help to exclude diabetes and syphilis as causes of the neuropathic joint. The poor vision makes one of the above likely.

Other causes of Charcot's joints include Charcot–Marie–Tooth syndrome, leprosy, syringomyelia and meningomyeloceles.

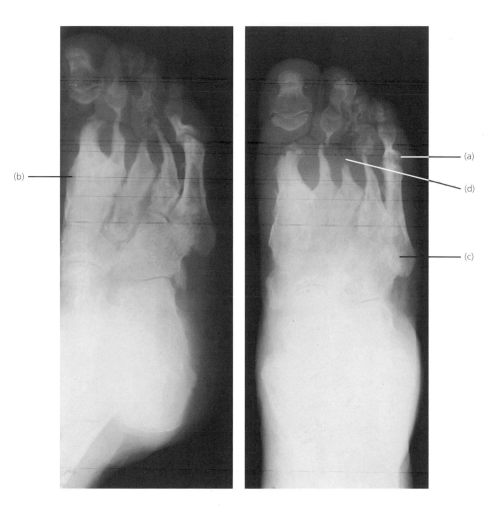

8

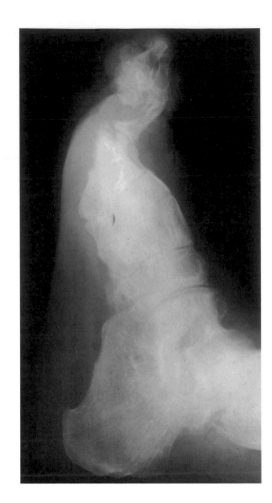

9

The X-ray of her hands shows (see opposite):
(a) soft-tissue swelling;
(b) ulnar deviation at the metacarpophalangeal joints;
(c) periarticular osteoporosis;
(d) loss of the joint spaces;
(e) erosion of the cartilage, particularly affecting the proximal interphalangeal joints, as well as:
(f) the metacarpophalangeal joints.

The diagnosis is rheumatoid arthritis. This is an inflammatory symmetrical arthritis which may lead to gross deformity of the hands. Swan neck and boutonnière deformity of the hands occur in addition to the deformities already mentioned. Wasting of the dorsal interosseous muscles together with the above lead to severe loss of function. Carpal tunnel syndrome is a common complication. The mainstay of management

9
for progressive disease involves prompt treatment with slow-acting antirheumatoid drugs (SAARDs) in order to reduce disease progression.

Severe disease is associated with certain HLA-DR4 subtypes in northern Europeans and Caucasians in particular. There are a number of extra-articular manifestations, which include vasculitis, leading to nail fold infarcts and multiple polyneuropathy (mononeuritis multiplex); eye involvement in the form of scleritis, episcleritis, scleromalacia and Sjögren's syndrome; neurological involvement due to atlantoaxial joint subluxation or a sensory neuropathy in a glove-and-stocking distribution; haematological manifestations in the form of anaemia, thrombocytopenia, neutropenia and splenomegaly (Felty's syndrome); respiratory involvement in the form of pulmonary fibrosis, pleural effusions, obliterative bronchiolitis and rheumatoid nodules; cardiac manifestations that include pericarditis, myocarditis and pericardial effusions; and renal failure may occur as a result of amyloidosis or analgesia nephropathy.

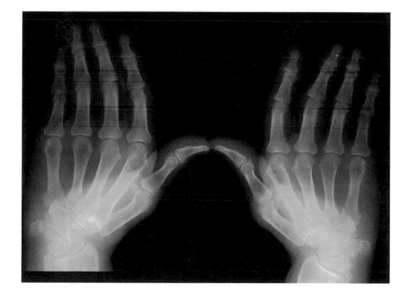

10
The Doppler scan of the femoral and popliteal veins would be negative in this case.

This is an arthrogram, which shows (see overleaf):
(a) extravasation of contrast outside the knee joint into the posterior aspect of the calf.

This is a ruptured Baker's cyst. Management involves rest and splinting of the knee, together with intra-articular steroid injections. Anticoagulation is not indicated. The patient is suffering from rheumatoid arthritis.

10

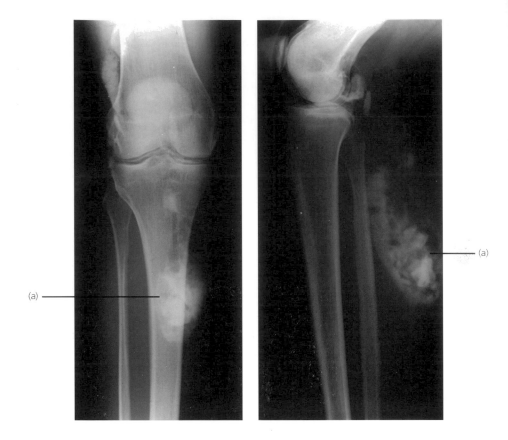

(a)

(a)

11

The X-ray shows (see opposite top):
(a) destructive punched-out lesions in the joint.
(b) tophi

These are typical of changes seen secondary to urate deposition. The cause of the pain is therefore gout.

This man has Lesch–Nyhan syndrome, which consists of mental retardation, self-mutilation and gout. This results from the deficiency of the enzyme hypoxanthine-guanine phosphoribosyl transferase, leading to an accumulation of purines, which are ultimately converted to urate. These strongly negatively birefringent crystals are deposited in the first metatarsophalangeal joint in about 70% of cases of gout. Chronic deposition leads to a reduction in the joint space, with subarticular punched-out lesions (chronic tophaceous gout). Soft-tissue calcification may also be visible. The acute condition is treated with colchicine or NSAIDs, and later with allopurinol while prophylactic anti-inflammatory therapy continues.

11

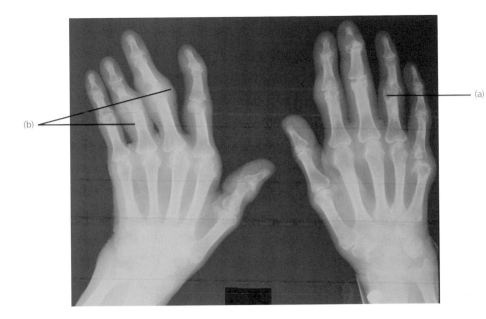

12

The ⁹⁹ᵐTc methylene diphosphonate (MDP) scan shows:
(a) areas of increased uptake of the isotope throughout the skeleton.

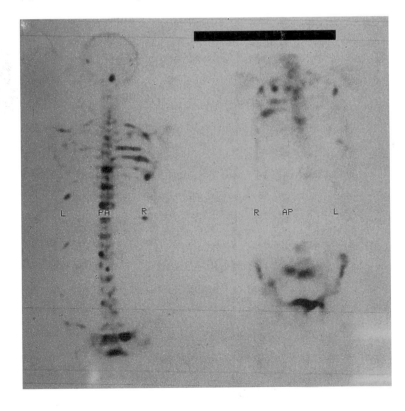

The diagnosis is metastatic carcinoma of the lung. Recurrent pneumonia in the same territory makes an obstructive lesion of the bronchi likely. Other locations of tumours that commonly metastasize to bone are the prostate, breast, thyroid and kidney.

13

The X-ray shows:
(a) obliteration of the sacroiliac joints.

This is a seronegative arthropathy secondary to inflammatory bowel disease. This man either has Crohn's disease or ulcerative colitis. Inflammation of axial and peripheral joints does not reflect intestinal disease activity.

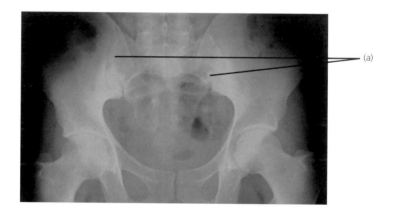

14

The X-ray shows (*see opposite*):
(a) periosteal elevation with new bone;
(b) bone lucencies;
(c) sclerosis.

These are typical appearances of osteomyelitis.

The likely cause is *Salmonella*, which is the commonest infective organism in sickle-cell disease. (The recent history of food poisoning would also help to support the diagnosis.)

Predisposing conditions leading to osteomyelitis are diabetes mellitus, intravenous drug abuse, sickle-cell disease, chronic urinary tract sepsis, diverticular disease, malabsorption and immunosuppression.

14

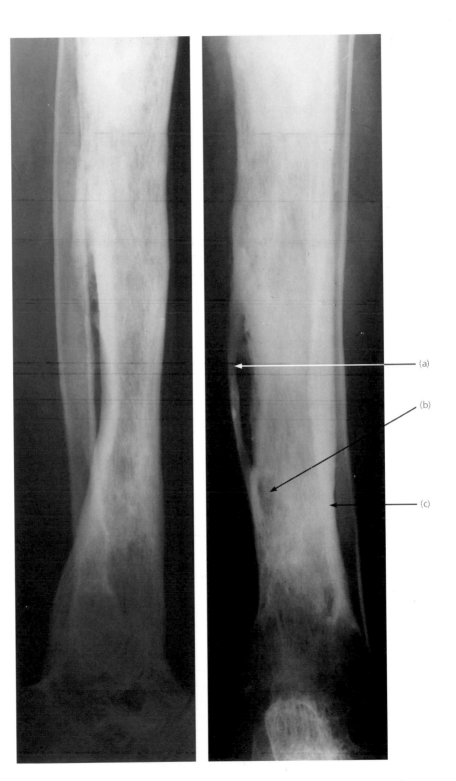

(a)

(b)

(c)

15

The spinal X-ray shows (see below and opposite):
(a) thinning of the cortex;
(b) a reduction in bone density;
(c) wedge collapse of T12 and L1;
(d) loss of disc height and sclerosis at the L5–S1 level.

These appearances are typical of osteoporosis. The physical appearance described in the question, together with infertility and osteoporosis in a young man, suggests hypogonadism secondary to Klinefelter's syndrome. Chromosomal analysis will confirm a 47 XXY genotype, and seminal fluid examination will confirm azoospermia. Treatment with testosterone injections will reduce the chance of further osteoporosis.

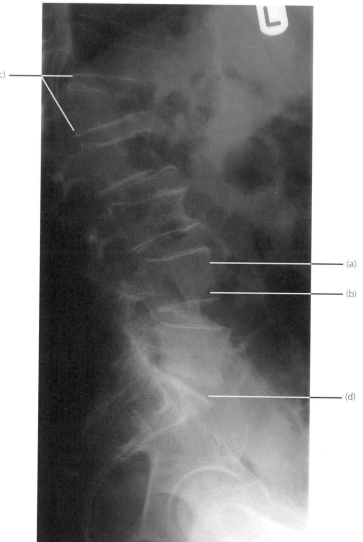

15

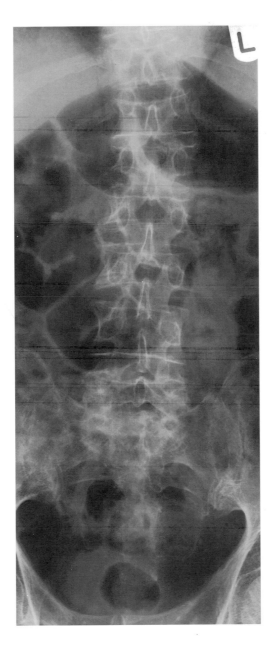

16

The X-rays show (see overleaf):
(a) calcification of subcutaneous tissue;
(b) calcification of the muscle.

The diagnosis is dermatomyositis. Relevant testing should be done for muscle enzymes, a muscle biopsy should be taken, and electromyography (EMG) should be carried out. It is mandatory to exclude an underlying malignancy which occurs in around 10% of cases over the age of 50. Relevant tests include CXR, gastroscopy, colonoscopy and Ba studies.

16   Clinically, patients present with a proximal myopathy. On examination, there is facial oedema (especially periorbital) and a rash (heliotrope rash) over the dorsum of the hands and the extensor surfaces (Gottron's sign). Other systems may be involved, leading to myocarditis, pulmonary fibrosis and dysphagia. Treatment is with high-dose steroids and immunosuppression.

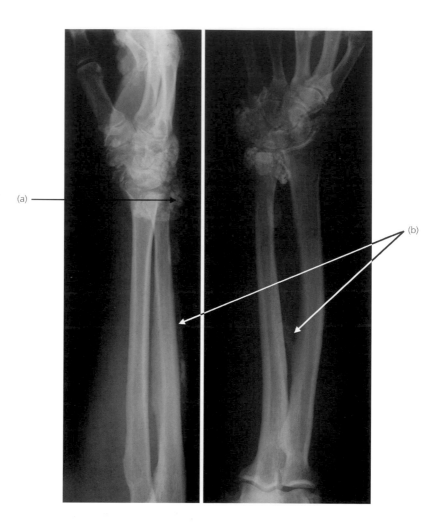

17   *The X-ray shows*:
(a) calcification of the voluntary muscles at the elbow joint (brachialis).

The diagnosis is myositis ossificans. Repeated trauma of the same voluntary muscle groups may give rise to this appearance. Progressive myositis

17

ossificans is an autosomal dominant disorder, characterized by sclerosis of the intramuscular connective tissue and subsequent ossification. Muscles of the back, shoulder and pelvic girdle are involved.

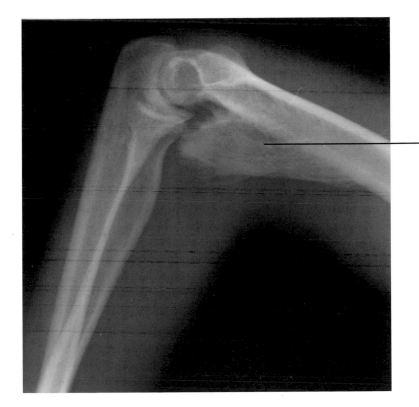

18

The X-ray of the tibia shows (see overleaf top):
(a) periosteal new bone formation in the tibia and fibula.

This is hypertrophic pulmonary osteoarthropathy (HPOA).

The X-ray of the left shoulder shows (see overleaf bottom):
(b) lytic destruction of the humerus due to metastasis.

A CXR should be done, which will show (see p. 341):
(c) a pulmonary mass consistent with bronchogenic carcinoma (shown by arrowheads).

New bone formation (in HPOA) occurs in the long bones, typically at the wrists and ankles. Bone metastases are common. Other skeletal manifestations of bronchial neoplasms include lytic lesions due to secretion

18

of PTH-related peptide, and osteoporosis due to ectopic secretion of adrenocorticotrophic hormone (ACTH).

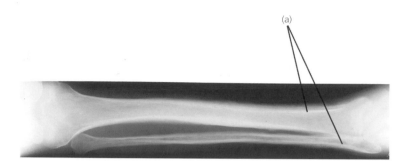

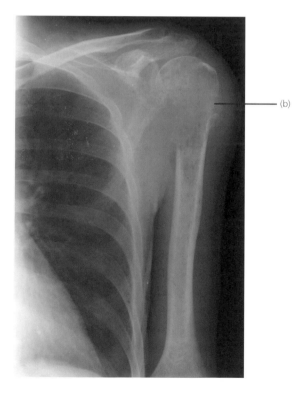

18

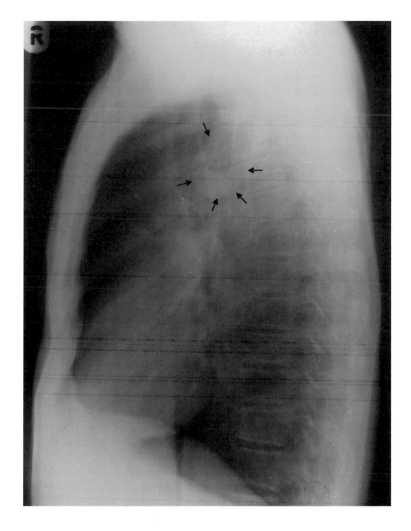

Index